Inspiration PRN: Stories About Nurses

A Collection of Spiritual Lessons

By

David S. Gerstle, Ph.D., R.N.
&
Bonnie C. Hunt, M.S.N., R.N.

© 2003 by David S. Gerstle, Ph.D., R.N. &
Bonnie C. Hunt, M.S.N., R.N. All rights reserved.

No part of this book may be reproduced, stored in a retrieval system, or transmitted by any means, electronic, mechanical, photocopying, recording, or otherwise, without written permission from the author.

ISBN: 1-4107-8266-2 (e-book)
ISBN: 1-4107-8267-0 (Paperback)

This book is printed on acid free paper.

1stBooks - rev. 09/30/03

Photo credits: David S. Gerstle, Bonnie C. Hunt

Photo Models: Steve Cash, Laura David

Dedicated

To nurses of the past,

To practicing nurses,

To future nurses, and

To friends of nurses.

Preface

Fifteen years of my nursing career has been spent in clinical practice in hospitals and home health agencies in a variety of roles. I have worked as a staff nurse, charge nurse, unit manager, nursing supervisor, and as a director of medical-surgical nursing services in hospitals. I have been a staff home health nurse and case manager in addition to my hospital experience. For the past nine years, I have taught in a school of nursing. The idea of writing this collection of short stories about nursing was formed when I began to realize that my nursing experience had provided me with many spiritual lessons. As I taught students, I would share some of these experiences with them. It was then that I was convinced that these stories and their lessons should be written in a book to share with others.

David S. Gerstle, Ph.D. R.N.

After teaching in a school of nursing for 20 years, I continued my teaching role in my retirement as co-coordinator of an assisted learning program, Assisting Students to Achieve Professionally (ASAP). During my years of teaching, I also worked in a local hospital as a staff nurse to keep up my nursing skills. It was during this time that I became aware how misunderstood is the role of the nurse. Improving the image of nursing became my passion. The opportunity to share that passion through writing inspirational stories about nurses has been an interest of mine for several years.

Bonnie C. Hunt, M.S.N., R.N.

Table of Contents

PRAYER...A MUST 1
Jesus Prays With Us 3
Near Misses 6
"Can We Pray?" 9
Atheist Prayer 11

JUST A NURSE? 17
Just a Nurse? 19
Just a Nurse...Same Song Second Verse 22
CATs, PETs, and MRIs Don't Supply the Care; 24
Nurses Do 24
Life is Backwards 26
No Brains, All Brawn 29
The Name is Nurse. Male Nurse! 34

KINDNESS - GOOD WILL TO ALL 37
Ministry of a Meal Ticket 39
There's Room for One More 43
Too Busy to Help? 45
First Clinical Jitters 47
Gifts Differing 50

Having Done It for One of the Least 52
The Return of Christmas Gifts 54
Singing Nurse Assistant 57

SPIRITUAL LIFE—FIRST THINGS FIRST 61
A Bedpan by Any Other Name... 63
Windy Wake-Up Call 66
Living Water 68
Good Medicine 70
The Healing Word 73
Christmas Code Blue 76
Dismayed 82
Unusual? Maybe Not 84
Promises 86

NEVER GIVE UP 89
Never Give Up! 91
Never, Never, Never, Never, Give Up 94
The Virtue of Observation 98
Disillusioned 100
Body Image Aerobics 103
Ain't Gonna Do It! 109
Florence 113
A Train with No Caboose 116

PERCEPTIONS ... 119
Knifepoint ... 121
Jumping to Conclusions ... 125
You Know I (Can) Dance ... 130
Instructions ... 133
Don't Run ... 135

COMFORT MEASURES ... 137
Painful Lessons ... 139
How Will I Know I'm Hurting? ... 142
Painful Confusion ... 145
Solving the Wrong Problem ... 150
A Shoulder to Cry On ... 152
Out of the Darkness ... 154
CCU Madness ... 159
Left to Die ... 163
The Way Home ... 167
Plans ... 169

"O DEATH, WHERE IS THY STING?" ... 171
"Though I walk through the valley ... 173
of the shadow of death..." ... 173
A New Beginning ... 178
Will to Live, Will to Die ... 181

GETTING ALONG…LET'S TRY IT	187
Why Can't We Play Nice?	189
Fight, Fight!	193
THE DUFF'S - A FAMILY AFFAIR	197
The Duffs	199
Guardian Angel	200
Doing What Is Right	203
God's Answer	205
While the World Partied	208
God I Need You Again!	211
Another Guarding Angel	212
ACKNOWLEDGMENTS	217

Inspiration PRN: Stories About Nurses

PRAYER...A MUST

Jesus Prays With Us

Have you ever seen the paintings in which a nurse or physician is standing at the bedside, praying for the patient? This scene seems to imply that patients are the recipients of the prayer and are not sharing in the prayer for their own healing or safety. It communicates the idea that the person providing care is the one who alone offers up these petitions to God on behalf of the one suffering. This perception of mine was shattered one day when I worked on a busy hospital surgical unit. The clerk in the surgery department called the floor and asked that Mr. Clark be given his pre-operative medications for his back surgery that was scheduled that morning. Mr. Clark was assigned to Joan, another RN working with me that day. I went down the hall to find her and let her know that Mr. Clark needed to be prepared for surgery. I had just seen her in the vicinity of Mr. Clark's room so I headed in that direction. I passed by his door and noticed that it was slightly open. Peeking inside, I saw Mr. Clark and Joan kneeling together in prayer beside his bed. I slowly backed away not wanting to disturb them for I knew that their prayers were much more important at this time than the preoperative medication. Leaving the door open just a little, I quietly stood there in awe of what was quietly happening at the bedside of this preoperative patient. The elderly man and the nurse together on their knees, were bowing before God, asking Him to guide the surgeon's hands in the operating room. What struck me so intensely was that the nurse was not standing beside the bed praying for the patient, but was clasping the hands of the patient and kneeling with him as his prayer partner. In turn, the nurse and the patient talked with their Lord in the small private patient's room on a busy surgical floor, seemingly oblivious of their surroundings. Divinity and humanity for a moment in time linked in conversation asking for help from the Heavenly Father.

    If I could only paint; I would create a new rendition of the patient and the nurse in prayer. I would paint what I saw that morning. The patient and nurse on their knees together. Of course, we nurses know most of our patients are so ill or injured they cannot get on their knees literally. Yet what this picture symbolizes is so important. The significance of the nurse and patient praying together is powerful. Not only is it a petition brought before God to bring safety, healing, and comfort, but also the act of praying together brings the patient into the circle of communicating with God as an equal partner with the nurse in seeking a return to wellness. Together, the patient and the nurse pray to God the Father, abiding in faith that the gift of healing will be given.

    There is something even more powerful than the patient and nurse praying together. Our Savior, Jesus, also prays with us when we pray. Phillip Samaan, professor of religion at Southern Adventist University says, "Jesus wants to be our prayer partner. He wants to pray for us." Hebrews 7:25 states, "Wherefore He is able also to save them to the uttermost that come unto God by Him; seeing He ever lives to make intercession for them." A quote from the book, *The Desire of Ages* states "Jesus lives to pray for us. In the Garden of Gethsemane, Jesus wanted His disciples to pray with Him, but they slumbered on. After His death and ascension, Jesus explained to his disciples that "He would be present before the Father to make request for them. The prayer of the humble suppliant He presents as His own desire in that soul's behalf. Every sincere prayer is heard in heaven. It may not be fluently expressed; but if the heart is in it, it will ascend to the sanctuary where Jesus ministers, and He will present it to the father without one awkward, stammering word, beautiful and fragrant with the incense of His own perfection."[1]

What an awesome thought it is that Jesus joins the nurse and patient in prayer. How can one ever feel that prayers are not heard when Jesus is offering the same prayers and presenting them to the Father? The next time you are discouraged or feel that your prayers go unheard, remember Jesus is praying for you and with you. Invite your patients to pray with you and let them know Jesus is your prayer partner.

David Gerstle

Near Misses

The memory of the incident still haunts me. Christy Hayes, a student nurse, had just received report on her patients when surgery called and said they were coming to pick up one of Christy's patients. Since this was the students' first day for this particular rotation, I assisted Christy with preparing Mrs. Eaves, the patient, for surgery. We dashed around checking to see if the permit was signed and the lab work was on the chart. Christy drew up the pre-op medication, then checked for nail polish and make-up and had Mrs. Eaves empty her bladder. The orderly appeared at the door with the gurney, so Christy quickly administered the pre-op medication. Then it was with frightened eyes that the patient looked at us and asked, "Are you Christians?" We both replied "yes" and she said "pray for me quick!" Startled Christy and I shamefully looked at each other. Quickly regaining our composure, Christy offered a prayer for the patient's safety in surgery and a quick recovery. Thanking us for the prayer and looking somewhat relieved, Mrs. Eaves was rolled out of the room on the gurney and down the hall to surgery. After talking with the family for a few minutes and still feeling a little awkward over the incident we hastily exited the room.

"I hope I don't ever do that again...be so busy doing the one, two three's, of my duties and overlook the patient's need for me to pray with them", groaned Christy. I told Christy I too felt sad that we had not sensed Mrs. Eaves need for spiritual care.

It had been one of those shifts that one tends to think will never get under control...a fresh surgery patient's blood pressure dropping precipitously, another patient's temperature rising to 104.2 with blood cultures to be drawn and then STAT antibiotics, a chemotherapy patient accidentally pulling out her IV line, plus two new admissions. I only had time for a hasty check here and there on Mrs. Hawkins as she lay there alone in her room. She was quiet except for an occasional moan as she drifted in and out of a semi-stuperous state. It was the end of the shift and I was still feeling rushed and frustrated. I was tempted to quickly clear Mrs. Hawkins's IV pump and empty her foley and then be on my way; but the incident with Christy flashed through my mind. A saying I had read for my devotion that morning popped into my head, "you can always pray for someone when you don't have the strength to help him in some other way". I knew I had to take the time to comfort her. "Mrs. Hawkins would you like for me to pray for you?" I whispered in the ear of this frail dying elderly lady. To my surprise she opened her eyes and nodded her head. "Dear Jesus, send comfort, peace and a good night's rest for this precious soul." Voice cracking, I continued. "May she rest in the promise that you will be with her always. Amen". During the prayer Mrs. Hawkins started to sob uncontrollably. I held her hand and patted her shoulder trying to comfort her. The sobbing went on for quite some time. I began to wonder if I had done more harm than good. Finally, the sobbing quieted. Feeling distressed that I might have caused her more grief, I left the room. Later Mrs. Hawkins' family told me that after I prayed, Mrs. Hawkins told them she drifted off in a more peaceful sleep and rested better that night. A few days later she slipped into a coma and died.

Sue Allen, a nursing instructor, and a student went to remove a naso gastric feeding tube from Mrs. King, a patient who seemed to now tolerate oral nourishment. Mrs. King had a malignancy and had endured many painful and unpleasant procedures. After the student explained what she was going to do, Mrs. King looked up at Sue and pleaded "Oh pray it won't

Inspiration PRN: Stories About Nurses

hurt'. Quietly Sue took Mrs. King's hand, closed her eyes, and bowed her head briefly. After a moment she opened her eyes to see Mrs. King's eyes fixed on her. "That was an awfully short prayer," complained Mrs. King. Gently squeezing Mrs. King's hand, Sue whispered, "God hears short prayers too!" The naso gastric tube was removed without difficulty.

Months later Sue was "making rounds" when she entered the room of Mrs. King who had been readmitted to the hospital. Sue hardly recognized her...the cancer had taken its toll for there lay Mrs. King with a large swollen abdomen; her arms and legs where just "skin and bones". Surprised to see Sue, Mrs. King summoned a weak smile and then asked Sue if she would pray for her again. "I would like to do just that," responded Sue. Tearfully Sue asked God to bring comfort and peace to Mrs. King. Opening her eyes this time Sue saw Mrs. King slowly and with great effort raise her emaciated arm and hand and then she gently patted Sue on the check.

In recent years faith, prayer and illness has been of interest to researchers. One conclusion is that prayer has obvious appeal; it is easy-to- use, inexpensive, and has no apparent side effects. Even skeptics conclude that it won't hurt to try. Prayer can give hope and encouragement while reducing anxiety.

Holy Scriptures commands us to "Pray without ceasing" to "Pray one for another" and then rewards us with the promise that "The fervent prayer of a righteous man has tremendous power" James 5:16.

Bonnie Hunt

"Can We Pray?"

"Can we pray?" "Oh my yes! In the confusion of the moment I almost forgot. I am so thankful you remembered," was my sheepish reply to Gina's request. Gina was just leaving my office to go to the testing center to take the NCLEX (national licensure exam) for nursing when several faculty and classmates (who had already taken the exam) stopped by to wish her well. There were lots of hugs and gleeful chatter as well as "you can do it" encouragements. During the summer I had tutored and mentored students preparing for this most important examination and had faithfully prayed with each one just prior to their taking the exam. Now here was Gina, who had been a special challenge, and I was about to forget the most important preparation of all...prayer.

Earlier in the summer Gina had commented she was trying to get her spiritual life back on track and felt that would help her depression. Gina had admitted having no motivation to prepare for NCLEX. She said she tried but couldn't even force herself to study. The only motivation she had was to come to my office for the several times a week study sessions. The first part of these "study sessions" consisted of her deploring the fact that she had no motivation and yet knew she had to prepare for the exam to be successful. The next part of the study session was me "nagging"..."Gina just force yourself to practice 50 questions in the morning and 50 questions in the afternoon and pretty soon you will become motivated to practice more." Then we would end the session by doing some practice questions together which indicated all the more her need for some earnest preparation.

I have a prepared sheet for the students to keep track of how many questions they practice and their scores. Session after session Gina would bring her sheet in which would indicate she had only done about 25 practice questions without any scores to brag about. All summer long Gina and I had prodded along...with me continuously encouraging her to do more practice questions. Gradually Gina did more review on her own increasing the number of practice questions and, yes, her scores improved. Now it was time for Gina to take the NCLEX.

The faculty has taken seriously the injunctions to "Always have a prayerful attitude"[1] and to "Pray for each other" and are encouraged that "The fervent prayer of a righteous man has tremendous power."[2] To communicate this philosophy on a practical level, the School of Nursing has made a practice of putting on a bulletin board the names of students with the scheduled dates and times of their NCLEX exam. On the date of a student's exam there is a special spot on the bulletin board for their name to be placed with the time of the exam. This very visible spot enables the faculty to view who is taking the exam and the time so they can say a special prayer for that student at that time. After receiving notice of their success there is a "congratulations" spot for their name which is cause for great rejoicing. The students know that we do this and say they are very comforted by this practice and state they feel this is one reason they have been successful on NCLEX. Sadly, Gina had to remind me of this commitment to especially pray for her at this most stressful time. After claiming God's promise to give wisdom to those that ask and asking for God to send a calming spirit on Gina, she left the office a little nervous but smiling and hopeful of conquering the challenge.

Gina was successful on her NCLEX..."fervent" prayer does have tremendous power.

Bonnie Hunt

Atheist Prayer

"I don't believe in God!" exclaimed the young female post-operative patient.

"In fact, if He *does* exist, I hate Him! Look at what He is doing to me." she continued.

"Why is this happening to me? I have been a good person all of my life. I don't deserve this."

The day before she had undergone a nephrotomy for kidney stone extraction for about the third time in her life. The stones formed in her body were too large to pass or even to extract by less invasive basket retrievals. Extracorporeal lithotripsy was not even a consideration. Both kidneys were involved and the surgeon left Penrose drains in each incision, which required frequent dressing changes.

Sara was born in Indonesia and had lived in the United States for the past eight years. Her family moved to Texas soon after they arrived in the country. About three years passed before Sara had her first bout with kidney stones. The doctors warned her that Texas was a part of the stone belt in America, which seemed to particularly affect people moving there from overseas. Sara was one of those unfortunate people whose metabolism led to frequent stone formation. Over the years, she became bitter about the torment and frequent medical procedures this caused.

I had been caring for Sara for the past three evening shifts on the renal unit where I had worked. I had cared for a lot of patients with chronic renal calculi formation, but her experience with this condition was the worst I had seen. Her physician was concerned with the scarring the stones and subsequent surgery were causing. He had discussed with her that loss of her kidneys was an eventual possibility.

I had developed a good rapport with Sara; at least she had quickly confided in me her frustrations and misery with her situation. The first evening she had shared with me that she was an atheist and she believed God was just a fantasy in peoples' minds. She reasoned that if this supposedly loving God was real, He wouldn't let people suffer.

"Sara, you say you don't believe in God, but you hate Him?" I asked her not in a challenging tone but one that sought greater understanding.

"I said *if* He existed, I hate Him. I don't think He is real."

"I believe He is real."

"Why?" she asked simply.

Being a person who depends more on logic than emotion to understand things, I explained that it made sense that God existed. His words of advice and wisdom in the Bible made sense. I had seen people change from a selfish demeanor to a loving and generous one simply by dedicating their lives to Him. Creation by a supreme being made much more sense than the theory of evolution. On a more personal note, I feel whole when my relationship with God is intact than when at times of discouragement and I do not approach God on a daily basis.

Sara was quiet as I gave my explanation. She seemed to listen intently but not to what I thought she would be more interested in hearing.

"You get discouraged?" she asked meekly.

"Sure I do. More often than I like to admit. But praying and reading the Bible helps me a lot."

She began to share with me how she felt and how her medical problems made her angry and out of control of her life. I listened as I changed her dressings and administered her IV medications. As she shared with me, she became angry all over again just thinking about her troubles. She ended this conversation exclaiming her disbelief in God again and then covering her head with the bed covers. I left the room quietly, thinking that I made her more upset than when I entered the room. As I checked on her throughout the rest of the shift, she only spoke as necessary to be polite and nothing more. This confirmed my assumption about our first conversation.

The next evening I entered Sara's room fearing that she may not want to see me again after our last conversation. However, she greeted me with a slight smile and seemed to be in a happier mood. As I assessed her and cared for surgical incisions, she began her conversation again about how she did not believe in God.

"I don't believe in God, but last night you said you prayed to Him. How do you pray?"

"Well, it's nothing formal", I began, "I just talk to Him and tell Him about my problems. Like you would talk to a friend that you trust."

"How do you know He listens?"

"How do you know a friend listens?"

Sara contemplated this for a moment and then said, "I guess you feel that you are understood."

She paused and then added, "You feel accepted even when you are revealing your innermost emotions and limitations."

"That's how it can be with God if you get to know Him."

The conversation continued for a while as we talked about prayer. Sara asked more questions about talking to God and seemed intrigued. Yet, as we ended the conversation she stated again that she didn't believe in God. Towards the end of the shift, I made one final check on Sara; she was still awake and watching television.

"Sara, I'll see you tomorrow." I said as I began to leave the room.

"When you get home, you can pray for me."

The remark startled me and I asked Sara to repeat it.

She stammered a bit and said, "You know, you can pray for me to God. I don't believe in Him, but you can ask Him to heal me."

I assured her that I would do that for her.

This was the last evening that I would care for Sara before my week-end off. She was sitting in a chair when I came to her room. She seemed comfortable and greeted me with a little more enthusiasm than the evenings before.

"How are you doing, Sara?"

"You know, I feel better. The pain is less today and I have stayed up a lot longer than I have been doing."

She didn't bring up God as we talked about the care she would need to do for her incisions when she was dismissed from the hospital. The conversation was pleasant as I showed her what she needed to do.

Later that evening Sara turned on her call light and asked for me to come to her room. She wanted her water pitcher refilled. I left for the kitchen and returned with ice to add to the fresh water.

"You know I still don't believe in God." She stated matter-of-factly. "But, you do, so you can keep praying for me."

"I will certainly do that, Sara. But, are you sure you don't believe just a little bit in God?"

"I believe you believe."

Hesitantly she added, "And...I felt better last night knowing you prayed for me. If God does exist, He will hear your prayers for me."

I didn't see Sara again after that evening as she had been dismissed before I returned to work the next week. I don't know if she ever began to believe in God or began to pray on her own. I do know God wants everyone to believe in Him, yet He only wants it by the exercise of one's own free will. Words many times cannot convince, but actions and being an example can.

"But as many as received Him, to them He gave the right to become children of God, to those who believe in His name."[1]

David Gerstle

Inspiration PRN: Stories About Nurses

JUST A NURSE?

Just a Nurse?

The chemotherapy room was quiet except for an occasional beep from an infusion pump. Two patients were dozing in recliners, the third patient, Mrs. Watkins, was fidgeting in her purse for a "paper back" to read. Mr. Watkins was sitting quietly beside his wife watching intently the drip, drip, drip of his wife's first chemotherapy treatment. The morning had been busy for nurse Ruth Owens, assessing her patients, accessing their port-a-caths and starting their chemotherapy. She finally sat down to do the necessary paper work, but her eyes continued to sweep the room to check on her patients.

Suddenly a look of terror crosses Mrs. Watkins' face. She clasps her chest and utters, "I can't breathe." Her eyes roll back as her head slips to the side. Realizing her patient is having an anaphylactic reaction, Ruth leaps from her chair, presses the emergency button, discontinues the chemotherapy, slips an oxygen mask on Mrs. Watkins and wraps a blood pressure cuff around her arm. Almost immediately another nurse comes into the room and Ruth directs her to administer an antihistamine to stop the allergic reaction and cortisone to decrease the inflammation that is blocking the airway. Before the emergency team arrives, Mrs. Watkins' breathing returns to normal and the look of terror fades. Then Ruth turns to the three ashen faced onlookers and says quietly, "It's frightening to see something like this. But it is under control." Still shaken but with the color returning to his face, Mr. Watkins returns to the chair beside his wife and looks at Ruth inquiring "Are you a doctor?" "Oh no! I'm just a nurse," replies Ruth.

"We need a nurse in room 202," a nursing assistant calls the nurses' station. Nurse Jim Hewitt hurries down the hall to room 202 and finds Mrs. Green diaphoretic and saturated in perspiration from head to foot. Quickly assessing the situation, he asks her if she is diabetic. With a nod "yes" from Mrs. Green, Jim immediately obtains a low finger stick blood sugar...47. A call to the lab is placed. The tech says they are busy with an emergency but will come as soon as possible. After Mrs. Green drinks orange juice with added sugar, the finger stick blood sugar is repeated, 51. Several rounds of orange juice and 60 minutes later Mrs. Green's blood sugar is 79. Gown and bed linens changed, the lab tech finally arrives, and draws blood and calls back verifying the blood sugar is now 79. Checking to find the cause of Mrs. Green 's drop in blood sugar, Jim discovers she had her 5:30 p.m. NPH insulin but wasn't hungry so she did not eat her supper. "Any time you take your NPH insulin you must eat your recommended diet and also have a bed time snack," Jim reminds Mrs. Green. As Jim leaves the room the patient thanks Jim stating she feels a lot better and then admonishes, "Young man, why don't you go to medical school and become a doctor?"

    Members of "Southern Scholars" had gathered for a seminar class to discuss Virginia Wolfe's book *A Room of One's Own*. Spurned by the inequity of opportunities for female writers due to lack of financial independence and a place to create was Virginia Wolfe's inspiration for this book. She makes a compelling argument on the lack of encouragement and recognition that women receive for their talents and accomplishments particularly in the literary world. Even though the book was written in the early part of the twentieth century it was chosen to center the discussion on issues that face women in today's society. I was asked to moderate the discussion. While waiting for the seminar to begin, the students' conversation centered on what they would be doing after their upcoming graduation. A senior nursing student responded to the question what she planned to do with,

"Well, I am not going to be 'just a nurse'." Astonished at her reply and in the light of the topic for this particular discussion, I blurted out, "There is no such thing as 'just a nurse'!"

There are 2.2 million nurses making a significant impact on health care. A recent American Nurses Association slogan "Every patient needs a nurse" reflects the need for nurses in society. When asked whom they trust most of the health care professions, the public rates nursing highest. A survey on who the public perceives as the most "honest" of all professions (not just health care), nurses were rated number one, pharmacist number two, physicians number four and I'll let you guess who was rated last.

And let us not forget that Jesus' ministry was not only to preach the gospel but also to bring comfort and healing to the brokenhearted and the suffering. Since it is "nursing care" that brings about healing, I like to think of Jesus as a community health nurse for He went about Galilee..."preaching in the open air and healing people of every kind of sickness."[1] Also the apostle Paul reminds us, "There are different ways of serving the Lord, but all the gifts are given to honor Him..."It's true that there are different (spiritual) gifts...(some) are given a special measure of faith; another is given the gift of *healing*; and so on—all are given by the Holy Spirit."[2]

We are not "just nurses"! It is a special spiritual gift.

Bonnie Hunt

Just a Nurse...Same Song Second Verse

A very dedicated, competent, accomplished Master's prepared nurse friend of mine told me about her husband complaining, "You might know a lot about nursing but not much else." A little embarrassed about how true that might be, brought to mind all the times a bunch of us nurses got together and all we talked about was nursing. Defensively, I boasted to myself.

"So-oo if we know only a lot about nursing and not much else, just look at all we do." I have long been an advocate for promoting the image of nursing by emphasizing the vital role of nurses in health care. Nurses catch errors before they can happen...nurses can take pulmonary artery pressures with one hand while comforting the patient with the other...nurses deliver babies...nurses hang out their shingle and have their own practices...nurses save lives. I could go on but you get the picture. Because of all the good we do, my friend's husband's complaint not only stirred up embarrassment but a bit of resentment. Intuitively, I knew we are much more then "just a nurse."

Then it happened! I felt vindicated. As I read a devotional book for women by women, I often would read the biographical sketch about the author of that day's devotional. Over time it struck me how many nurses contributed to this book and the variety of activities in which these nurses were involved. "Well!" I thought to my self, "Just look at what all these nurses "do" (interpreted as "know") beside nursing."

The short biographies of the nurses that contributed to just one years' devotional book reflected accomplishments far beyond the field of nursing. For instance, the hobbies they were involved in included but went beyond the usual assortment of gardening, travel, music, handwork, exercise, and reading. There were scuba divers, oil painters, musicians, writers, kayakers, wake boarders, rock climbers and this hobby amused me, feeding backyard lake inhabitants such as fish, duck, birds, and worms, quite a show of dedication to the environment. Several of the registered nurses held Master's degrees in a field other than nursing, such as religion, business, counseling and education. Many held leadership positions in various organizations. There were directors of Women's ministries and other church offices, as well as one who served on the executive committee for a Christian business and professional women's club. One contributor who is a case manager for the seriously mentally ill, in her spare time volunteers for the "Make-a-Wish" foundation, produces a monthly newsletter, handles public relations for a church and Kiwanis. Some home schooled their children, while another taught driver's education, and, of course, many assisted husbands in their careers.

The "writers" captured my attention. The majority of the nurses' biographies revealed there were serious writers among us...not just the ones that had contributed to the devotional book but also the ones that had been published in a variety of ways. Their accomplishments included contributions to church papers, newspapers, and magazines. One nurse had not only contributed to the publications just mentioned but had a recent book of miracle stories, answered prayers, and angel encounters published. Also, among the writers was an associate editor of a Christian woman's magazine and a poetess.

Even though my sampling of nurses was very, very, small I still want to say "See there, we are a lot more then 'just a nurse' and take seriously Ecclesiastes 9:10 "Whatever you do, give it everything you've got and enjoy it."

Bonnie Hunt

CATs, PETs, and MRIs Don't Supply the Care; Nurses Do

(The title and the following tribute to nurses were excerpted from an article by Linda Chitwood - source unknown.)

Josh was born limp, blue, and severely brain damaged. The only cry in the delivery room was the soft weeping of his mother, Mary, an illiterate, impoverished adolescent. Josh was admitted to an intensive care unit. "His crib was shadowed by the best medicine could offer, yet nothing could medicine offer this child. Revolutionary treatment, sophisticated monitors, talented doctors—they could do nothing for this child."

A nurse "orchestrated" the bonding between baby and mother. A nurse taught Mary to feed Josh through his stomach tube, since he could neither suck nor swallow. A nurse drew a sun and moon, showing when to give Josh his medicines. A nurse taught Mary suctioning and seizure management. A nurse tramped through the mud to an isolated clapboard shack to demonstrate formula preparation in a home without electricity or running water. A nurse comforted Mary when Josh died. A nurse arranged for the pauper's burial.

Ms. Chitwood chides "And you thought nurses just carried out doctors' orders." Then she continues with, "Thank a nurse for noticing that the doctor has been ordering IV potassium supplements but hasn't checked a serum level in days. Thank a nurse for averting a near disaster when different doctors ordered conflicting treatments. Thank a nurse for comforting a patient with one hand while measuring pulmonary artery pressures with the other. Thank a nurse for calming anxious relatives when no one wanted to fool with them. Thank a nurse for monitoring the patients all night while you slept soundly. Thank a nurse for explaining what the doctor didn't have time to."

Ms. Chitwood concludes her article by urging us not to..."forget it was a nurse who made a difference in Josh's life. Not a neurosurgeon, not a CAT scanner, but a nurse. Nurses give their love and their lives. Let's give them the respect they deserve."

Thank you Ms. Chitwood for being on our side.

Dr. Thomas, physician and author of the book *The Youngest Scientist*, writes of his high respect of nursing as a profession. An illness that required an extended hospital stay clued him into things about nurses that his physician friends did not know. For one thing, he says, "nurses hold the place (hospital) together." "The institution is held together, glued together, enabled to function as an 'organism' by the nurses and by nobody else. They spot errors before errors can be launched. It takes a confident, competent, and cheerful nurse in and out of the room on one chore or another through the day and night to bolster ones confidence that the situation is indeed manageable and not about to get out of hand."

He closes his chapter on nurses with "Knowing what I know, I am all for the nurses. If they want their professional status enhanced and their pay increased, if they ask for the moon, I am on their side."

Thank you Dr. Thomas for being on our side.

God is on our side too. He encourages, "Let's not become tired of doing good, for in time, we'll reap the spiritual harvest if we don't give up."[1]

Bonnie Hunt

Life is Backwards

Beep, beep, beep. It was Mrs. Merchant's TPN running low this time. It seemed every time I passed Mrs. Merchant's room a piece of her equipment would be calling for my attention. Earlier it was her PCA pump that needed a refill...then it was one of her infusion pumps that beckoned for a new bag of IV fluids...then it was time to switch piggy backs from IV antibiotics to Pepcid...then Reglan...then another antibiotic. Each time I entered her room, Mrs. Merchant would stir a little and through the haze of her illness peer at me. I would inquire as to how she was feeling and was there anything else I could do for her. Her reply would vary from, "I am not bouncing back from this surgery like I should." or, "I just feel too bad to know if I even need anything else."

Since Mrs. Merchant had been too ill and too weak to be ambulatory, her physician had ordered that this evening she must get out of bed and walk in the room. With a few "oooohs" and "ouch" moans she stood at the side of the bed and then walked a few paces in the room. Putting her back to bed, I tried to arrange the pillows and her position to make her as comfortable as possible. Washing my hands after emptying her bulging Foley catheter bag, I was off to check on my other patients and try to meet their needs before the end of the shift.

Beep, beep, beep. Oh no! Now one of Mrs. Merchant's infusion pumps was yelling "occlusion! occlusion!" I quietly entered the room and found she was lying on the tubing compressing the flow. As gently as I could, I coaxed the tubing free and started to clear the infusion pumps for the end of the shift, when Mrs. Merchant stirred again and peered at me. "Life is all backwards," she whispered. "How's that?" I responded.

"Look at the wages of football players and entertainers compared to nurses and teachers." Weakly, she continued. "Just think of the contribution that nurses and teachers make to society." Then she turned back to her comfortable side and seemed to drift off to sleep.

As I completed my responsibilities for the end of the shift, the phrase "life is all backwards" kept running through my mind. I thought to my self, "Yes, life is all backwards in many aspects of life and nurses certainly are not exempt from this backwardness."

An editorial in the *St. Paul Pioneer Press*[1] (2001) aptly pointed out this backwardness. It was entitled, "Wanted: Good pay for quite a few good nurses." It seems the Minnesota Nurses Association was asking to raise the base pay for full-time nurses to something more reasonable then their present status. Surprisingly the public seemed to think the wage increase was not merited and decided to voice their opinion with comments like "Nurses don't even know how good they've got it." An interesting notion in light that musicians had just voted to ratify a contract that would adjust a beginning violinist pay well above what nurses were asking; also, airline inspectors had just ratified an hourly pay rate well above a nurse's salary.

"Nurses don't even know how good they've got it." You can say that only if you know nothing about nursing the editorial pointed out and then went on to say, "Let's review the job description. Wanted: "A compassionate and highly skilled caregiver willing to work evenings, weekends and major holidays, solving stressful problems (i.e., life or death) in highly collaborative environment, risking repeated exposure to everything from hepatitis to HIV, and working with a patient population sicker than ever before. Heavy lifting, constant hand-holding and occasional housekeeping (blood, urine, etc.) required."

I think we would all agree that society does have some backward values. I don't often think about the inequities of nurses' pay scale (not to say we shouldn't give it more thought). However, after reading the *St. Paul Pioneer Press* job description of a nurse, I felt vindicated for having chosen such a lofty profession. In reflecting on our lofty profession and the "backward value" issue, a thought came to me...do we as nurses have our values backward? Do the demands of our career cause us to neglect the "first things first" value? "...make God's kingdom and His righteousness first in your life..."[2] "You should love the Lord your God with all your heart, all your soul and all your mind."[3]

Some years ago I remember reading a compelling thought in a day-by-day devotional book. The thought has stuck with me..."Men do not order God out of their lives. At least, not many. They are just so cluttered up with preoccupying business that they have no time or attention for Him. We become so absorbed in our daily routine that our relationship to God and His church is pushed aside. We serve God with our spare time. We attend divine worship when nothing interferes. The things we are doing may be all right and good—yet here the good becomes an enemy of the best."

Putting "first things first" is not the result of chance. Sometimes we have to ask God to provide the time for us to put "first things first." This commitment brings its own reward. The Bible tells us "Not to worry about what to eat or what to drink or what to wear."[4] If we make God and His kingdom first, all those things will be given to us as we need them.

Making God first is the secret to reversing the "life is all backwards" syndrome.

Bonnie Hunt

No Brains, All Brawn

I had just graduated from nursing school when I was hired as a staff nurse at a large city hospital. The unit I was assigned to was "in between head nurses" at the time. The senior charge nurse was the interim manager and was an excellent mentor to me. She helped me learn to organize my care, chart, and perform many procedures. She was particularly impressed with my newly found venipuncture abilities and so was I. I felt like a "real" nurse instead of a student nurse. I was feeling really good about my chosen profession, that is, until a new head nurse arrived.

Mrs. Palmer was the head nurse on another nursing unit. She had been a wonderful nurse for years at this hospital, but recently she was in constant conflict with her staff. Her interpersonal skills were somewhat similar to Attila the Hun's. The "powers-that-be" decided she needed a new environment. As a last chance opportunity to redeem her, they made her the head nurse on our floor.

Mrs. Palmer was a large woman and resented walking. I suppose she had done a lot of it over the many years she has been a hospital nurse. She preferred to sit in her office overlooking her new kingdom and her subjects. She would sit there most of the day and write care plans. (For the younger readers, yes, we actually wrote care plans in real life years ago.) Once in a while, the Queen would get up and make rounds on the patients. Most of the time, however, she would call you to her office to get the end-of-shift report. She would call the nurses' station and ask the unit clerk to page each nurse in turn. We were not allowed to give our own report. This was the head nurse's job. Staff nurses were not capable, except on Mrs. Palmer's days off, to give report. It was obvious from the beginning of her reign that she wanted to be in complete control of our unit.

One day, our new head nurse decided she would speak with every nurse individually and let each of us know how she was going to run "her unit." One by one, we were summoned to her office. Finally, it was my turn. Being a new RN and the only male on the shift, I was nervous. I entered Her Majesty's office and took a seat. It was explained to me that she ran a "tight ship" and that everything was going to be done right. There would be no room for error. OK, I was all for quality and I wanted to do a good job, although my lack of experience concerned me.

Then, she dropped a bomb on me:

"Since you are a male nurse (she strongly emphasized "male" and not in a complimentary way), you *do* realize you were hired for your brawn and not your brain!"

I was shocked. I think my mouth fell open which I know made me look very intelligent.

"You just do what I tell you and we'll get along just fine." Mrs. Palmer continued.

I was then dismissed. I crawled out of her office, not sure whether I should be angry or depressed.

Her "brawn not your brain" lecture got to me more than I realized. I began to lose my self-confidence. One way this exhibited itself was that suddenly I could not start IVs.

"Mrs. Palmer", I stammered, "I'm sorry to bother you, but I've tried to start this IV and I can't do it." (Gulp, gulp) "Everyone else is busy so I've come to ask you to help me."

I am sure even though she was sitting in her office, I must have suggested she wasn't busy. This was a big mistake!

"Humph!, I'm busy too!" She slammed down her pencil (She was probably writing another care plan).

"What's the matter with you? Where did you go to school? Why can't you start an IV?"

I stuttered and stammered, "I haven't had trouble before, but I just can't start this one."

She rolled her eyes and then bore a hole through my head as she stared at me with an angry frown.

"I'll do it when I'm done here," she said no longer looking at me and as she waved me away with her hand. I felt like an admonished child with no brain and now not even any brawn.

A while later, the Queen finds me and now has a big grin on her face. In a loud voice for all to hear, she announces:

"I started that IV *yooooou* couldn't start! It took me just one stick. I can't believe you couldn't start it!"

She then gave a loud cackle-like laugh to finish me off. I was completely humiliated.

Of course, each of the next IVs I attempted ended in failure also. On more than one occasion, I had to ask Mrs. Palmer for help and each time she went out of her way to embarrass me about it. Each time it took more confidence away from me.

This went on for a while. Other new nurses realized what was happening to me and they began to share what the new head nurse was doing to them. She was tormenting each about one thing or another, whether it was IVs, other procedures, or taking too long for breaks. We decided, "enough was enough" and went to the experienced charge nurses for help. They came to our rescue and reported these incidents. Soon, Mrs. Palmer was given another new environment. Having been a loyal employee in the past, administration allowed her to retire early since she was only months from it anyway.

Our next head nurse was an interim replacement while the senior charge nurse was groomed to be the permanent head nurse. Mrs. Benton was kind and understanding. She was also a beautiful woman and no

Inspiration PRN: Stories About Nurses

matter how bad her day she was always immaculate. She didn't sit in her office all day; she worked along side us lowly staff nurses.

Early on, Mrs. Benton decided to talk to each of us individually. Uh, oh, perhaps she is not what she appears. Maybe she worked with us to see what terrible nurses we were. My self-confidence was still lacking! My turn came and I sat down in the office fully expecting another all brawn and no brain lecture from this new head nurse. Maybe I was getting fired and needed to practice saying, "Would you like fries with that?" I had started an IV that morning, maybe that would save me from the inevitable dismissal. Maybe it wouldn't and I would be thrown out of the hospital as the entire staff gathered along the halls pointing fingers at me and saying, "No Brains couldn't even start an IV!" while they cackled and guffawed along with Mrs. Palmer. What an imagination; I needed to get over this!

"Hi, Dave." Mrs. Benton greeted me with a warm smile.

"Hello." I stammered.

"I understand you have really been given a hard time lately. I want you to know I really appreciate you sticking it out. I enjoy working with new nurses and I am going to make you a promise. I am going to take you under my wing and help you be the best."

This was sounding good so far.

"But," she continued.

Uh, oh, bad sign.

"This is how I am going to do it. I am going to assign you the most critical patients. I am going to throw every tube insertion, IV start, and any other procedure that comes along."

"But," she added.

Another "but"; I hope the brawn/brain lecture isn't surfacing again.

"I will help you whenever you need it. You can come to me anytime."

I was in shock again, but this time I didn't feel stupid. I felt my confidence returning.

She did exactly what she promised. I got the hardest patients and Mrs. Benton kept me busy with every kind of procedure ordered. It wasn't long before other nurses were asking me to start IVs for them. What a difference it made in me for the better when the head nurse took a *positive* interest in me and encouraged me. It was totally the opposite effect caused by the first head nurse who made every attempt to tear me down.

I learned a lot that first year of nursing. It helped me advance in my career and to realize what an influence one can have on others. Take time to help those around you. What a blessing you can be! New nurses look up to experienced nurses. Take the time to teach and encourage. It can only improve our profession as those helped will learn to do the same.

"Let us therefore come boldly to the throne of grace, that we may obtain mercy and find grace."[1]

David Gerstle

The Name is Nurse. Male Nurse!

"Why in the world would a *man* want to be a nurse?"

The old farmer, who was one of my patients, practically spit those words at me along with a mouthful of his lunch.

"Honey!" his wife shouted. "You be nice! He is taking good care of you."

"I know, I know, but I just don't understand it. It's women's work." Farmer Brown shot back.

His wife hit him with a rolled up newspaper.

Over my 24 years as a RN, I've been confronted with this viewpoint numerous times. When I first began my career, it really bothered me. It made me feel different or odd. A male nurse! How strange! It took a couple of years for me to feel comfortable in my new role as a RN. As I continued to care for patients, I soon found out I had something to offer and patients and their families really appreciated it. I found that as a man I could bring a different perspective to patient care. Male patients appreciated me because it saved them a lot of embarrassment. They don't have to be as "macho" since there isn't a female nurse around to impress. Two guys can form a brotherhood and work together as the care is given. Female patients many times appreciate male nurses as well. Male nurses can't form a sisterhood with them, but we can be protectors and providers.

Now, please understand I prefer being called a "registered nurse" over "male nurse." However, it doesn't bother me anymore when I am called a "male nurse." In fact, I carry it with pride. It's almost like being a special agent (like James Bond) for the profession of nursing. My mission is to open the borders of nursing even further to men. (Fellow "male nurses," it is your mission too, should you choose to accept it.)

Yes, my name is Nurse. Male Nurse.

Why would a man want to be a nurse? There are many reasons to choose from: 1. To belong to a humanitarian profession helping people throughout their illness or injuries, 2. To do something worthwhile serving others as Jesus did, 3. To lead other nurses in their practice as you gain experience, 4. To educate patients on more healthful living, and many others.

If you are a "male nurse," be proud and be a role model. Encourage other men who are looking for a rewarding career to investigate nursing. Be a 007. Go ahead, be a Nurse. Male Nurse.

"And whatever you do in word or deed, do all in the name of the Lord Jesus, giving thanks to God the Father through Him."[1]

David Gerstle

Inspiration PRN: Stories About Nurses

KINDNESS - GOOD WILL TO ALL
"A GOOD THING"

Ministry of a Meal Ticket

It is just made of paper and not much bigger than a business card. Each one is worth about $20 in the hospital cafeteria where I worked as a nurse. Different amounts are on the card: $1, 50 cents, 25 cents, 10 cents, 1 cent; each of which can be punched out as you make purchases of food. It was quite convenient to buy a meal ticket as a payroll deduction so that one didn't need to always worry about money for lunch or supper.

However, a meal ticket was not just a convenience for the person purchasing it, but could be turned into a blessing for others when it was shared.

Driving to the hospital early one morning, I stopped for gas at a truck stop in the little town I drove through every day. After filling my tank and paying for it, a young man in his twenties approached me and asked for a lift.

"Excuse me, but are you headed toward Interstate 35?"

"Yes, I work at a hospital near Fort Worth, so I can take you that far."

"Hey, that would be just great" he said as we both got in my truck and headed toward the hospital.

As we drove along, the hitchhiker shared with me his recent traveling. He was 20 years old and had lost direction in life, gotten in trouble, and had been thrown out of the house by his parents. His older sister said he could live with her in Houston until he got on his feet again. He had begun hitchhiking from Alabama; heading toward Houston. He had gotten a ride from a trucker who worked for McKee Foods, the makers of Little Debbie snack cakes. The trucker had called a friend who was traveling to Houston from Cleburne, Texas, that day and had asked him to pick him up at the truck stop early this

Inspiration PRN: Stories About Nurses

morning. For whatever reason, the friend did not show as scheduled and now the hitchhiker wanted to get to the interstate in order to have a better chance to hitch a ride to Houston, 250 miles south.

"Well, I'm sorry your ride didn't work out. Would you rather go by bus? I could get someone from the hospital to take you to the station."

"Naw, I don't have enough money."

He seemed a little embarrassed, so he changed the subject.

"What hospital do you work at?"

"Huguley Hospital, it's operated by the Seventh-Day Adventist Church. Have you heard of them?'

The hitchhiker sat silently for a moment and then said, "The trucker who picked me up was a Seventh-Day Adventist. He said his company was owned by an Adventist. This is really weird, getting rides from two Adventists."

He paused for a moment and then said, "Maybe God is trying to tell me something. I haven't been in a church since I was a kid."

"Well, He may be." I said. "He does work in mysterious ways."

We reached the hospital and walked into the lobby.

"Have you had any breakfast?" I asked.

"No, but that's ok. I need to start hitching a ride anyway."

"Well, listen, I'll take you down to the cafeteria. I have an idea about how to get you to Houston. Here's my meal ticket; you get whatever you want. I need to check with the supervisor that I am relieving and then I will come get you."

After letting the other house supervisor know what was going on, I got on the phone and called the head deacon of my church. Since I was the community services leader, I asked him to bring some cash for food and a bus ticket to Houston and take my newfound friend to the Fort Worth bus station. Steve, the head deacon, was a wonderful and generous person and replied he would be there soon. I went down to the cafeteria and sat with the hitchhiker until Steve arrived. I explained to him that my church was capable of helping him get to his destination and that we would get him on a bus to Houston.

Somewhat shocked, the hitchhiker says, "You really don't have to do that."

About this time, Steve arrives with a big smile on his face and a Bible in his hand. After introductions, Steve says, "We are glad to have a chance to help you get to where you are going. In fact, I brought you something to read on your trip." as he hands him the Bible. "Reading this book has always helped me when I was facing big changes in my life."

The hitchhiker looked at the book and then at me and said, "God really must be trying to tell me something."

I told him goodbye as they got in Steve's car.

"Thanks for breakfast and for getting me to Houston. It will be a new beginning for me." as he held up his new Bible.

The quiet ministry of a meal ticket.

Karen was the charge nurse on the evening shift. One of her patients had severe fractures to his leg from an industrial accident and had to have emergency surgery. He would be in the hospital several days. Karen noticed after the first two evenings that the patient's wife brought her two young children to visit around suppertime. She saw that the children would have a bag of chips or some other snack food from a vending machine, and the mother would not be eating anything. Karen, when she was in the room, overheard the children saying they were hungry and wanted more to eat. The mother would just quiet them and tell them that the snacks were all they could have. Becoming concerned,

Inspiration PRN: Stories About Nurses

Karen asked the mother what was going on and she told her that with her husband being injured, they had lost all of their income suddenly. She was trying to keep up on the bills, so food was hard to afford. She had no one to care for the children, so she would bring them with her to the hospital.

Karen knew that Social Services could help them, but until all of the paperwork went through, there would be no money for food. Karen quietly slipped her new meal ticket into the mother's hands.

"Use this meal ticket in our cafeteria to get something to eat."

The quiet ministry of a meal ticket.

Don, a brand new nurse working on the night shift, was having a hard time adjusting to a new job and night hours. Feeling depressed, he was considering quitting nursing all together. The past several days he did his job, but his peers working with him knew he was struggling. The night charge nurse, Ann, after a tough shift, invited Don to breakfast.

"Don, you worked hard tonight. Breakfast is on me; I have plenty on my meal ticket."

They sat together, a young new nurse and a mature veteran of the night shift. They shared the tough times and the nice times. Ann was able to convince Don that things do get easier and that nursing can be very gratifying. Because of a meal ticket, two nurses, novice and expert, had an opportunity to salvage a nurse's career. The quiet ministry of a meal ticket.

David Gerstle

There's Room for One More

"Why is that grave marker in grandpa's cemetery plot? Who is it?"

It was a startling discovery for my wife, Nettie, while she was visiting her family in the piney woods of east Texas. She had not noticed the grave marker when she had visited her grandpa's grave as a child. But, there it was, a small marker with a name no one recognized. The dates on the marker revealed that the person died as an infant some years back.

"We'll ask Grandma when we visit her this afternoon." Nettie remarked.

My wife, her sister, and their mother placed some fresh flowers on Grandpa's grave and then drove to visit Grandma and ask about the mysterious grave marker.

Grandma Maudie was 88 years old and had been a nurse for years prior to her retirement. She had spent most of her time working as a private duty nurse. She also worked at the local nursing home. Maudie had a big heart and loved to help people whenever and wherever she could. In addition to her nursing career, she cared for many foster children. She was active in her church and well known in the small rural community where she lived. Everyone knew and trusted Maudie.

"Grandma, we visited Grandpa's grave today. Whose is the other grave marker in the family cemetery plot?"

"Oh, that's a baby buried there."

"OK." my wife said slowly, attempting to analyze that simple answer, "Uh, whose baby?"

"Honey, there was this poor family that lived nearby and their baby died after a long illness. They just didn't have any money to bury the little thing." Grandma explained.

"I told them there was no need to worry about buying a plot; they could just put their baby next to Grandpa. There's plenty of room left for me and that little baby."

That was typical of Grandma. As a nurse and as a caring person, Maudie always made room for one more, whether it was a spot in a cemetery plot, or a place for a foster child to stay, or another mouth to feed at her table. She always had room in her heart to care for one more.

Is there room for one more in your heart? Are you generous when it comes to helping others? Nursing is a caring profession, yet from time to time, we feel overtaxed in caring for those around us. The Bible tells us to love our neighbors and do good. Sometimes when we feel low and uncared for ourselves, doing something nice for another will uplift our spirits and make us feel good. It certainly benefits those we help. So, be generous and make room in your life to help others.

As Maudie says "There's room for one more!"

David Gerstle

Too Busy to Help?

In addition to being knee deep into a family nurse practitioner program, Laura and Bodil were working full time and had family responsibilities. Frequently they rode to class to gather chatting about their work or their family or the class they were taking. And often they would pray together asking God to help them not to be so consumed with their plight that they neglect to help someone in need.

Driving to class one afternoon, Laura and Bodil were somewhat preoccupied discussing the upcoming pharmacology class and their soon to be responsibility of prescribing drugs. The truck in front of them was slowing them down and they did not want to be late for class. Even though it was just a two-lane road Laura looked for a single yellow line in hopes of passing the truck. Then she noticed that the driver of the truck would slump to the right of the stirring wheel and then lean way over to the left of the wheel. He kept swaying back and forth as he drove ahead of them. Laura shouted "Bodil! Look at that man in the truck, I think something is wrong with him!" About that time the truck started to cross the yellow median line into oncoming traffic.

Laura "laid" on her car horn in hopes of alerting the driver of the truck of the danger and to warn oncoming traffic. The truck slowly drifted back in his lane, but now the driver seemed to slump down onto the seat. Again the truck started to move erratically from lane to lane. Laura stayed very close behind the truck continuing to blow her horn. The driver would lift his head every so often but this did not stop his scary behavior. A tunnel was just around the bend and Laura knew that if something wasn't done soon this was a tragedy waiting to happen. Silently praying for guidance,

Inspiration PRN: Stories About Nurses

Laura pulled out crossing the median line ever so slightly frantically blowing her horn and flashing her lights to warn the oncoming traffic and still try to get the driver's attention.

Miraculously, just before entering the tunnel the truck drifted to the right shoulder of the road and after bumping about a bit came to a halt in a ditch.

Laura pulled in behind him. Bodil ran to call for help, as Laura rushed up to the driver's side of the truck. She opened the door and asked the man what was wrong. He muttered, "I'm diabetic." and then slumped motionless on the seat of the truck.

Laura remembered there were some Oreo cookies in her car. She ran back to her car and grabbed a hand full of cookies. Splitting the cookies in half, she wiped the white filling onto her finger and then rubbed it around the gums of this motionless man.

Soon the police arrived and called for the paramedics. After transferring the man to the rescue vehicle, the paramedics started an IV and rushed him to the hospital. Satisfied the man was in good hands, Laura and Bodil continued on to class.

Unfortunately the "busyness" of our life too often preoccupies us with our own needs that we neglect reaching out for others. Like Laura and Bodil, we need to pray that we are not so self absorbed that we do not respond to someone in need.

"When you who have possessions see a brother or sister in need but you don't help him, how can you say that you love God?"[1]

Bonnie Hunt

First Clinical Jitters

"Can you be excited and scared to death at the same time? The answer is 'yes' for it happened to me," exclaimed Melita as she told me the story of her very first nursing school hospital clinical. "I set my alarm in time to get up early so I would have time to shower, dress with everything tucked in and in its proper place and eat a good breakfast in preparation for my first hospital clinical experience. As I settled in for a good night's sleep, I checked the alarm again and assuring it was properly set. When I snuggled so 'comfy' under the covers, I began to yawn, hoping to drift into a much needed sleep. Instead of sweet sleep, I tossed and turned; throwing the covers off because I was too warm, and then yanking them back up because I was chilled. About every hour I checked the time to make sure the alarm was still set. I felt as if 'fear' was vying for the 'excitement' of tomorrow's events. I was so excited about going to the hospital to put into practice what I had learned, but still worried over would I really be able to put into practice what I had learned in all those on-campus labs. Would I really be able to bathe and change the bed linens while the patient assigned to me remained in bed? Would I administer the right medicines at the right time? Would my patient like me? I guess this was a classic case of first clinical jitters.

When the alarm finally went off at 5:00 a.m., I literally jumped out of bed. Feeling less than rested, I attempted to eat breakfast. I chewed my Cheerios just enough so that I could swallow them without choking. Now it was time for me to don the uniform I had been so eager to wear. Oh no! I muttered to myself as my heart sank...there hanging in the closet was my new 'wrinkly' uniform. In my excitement of the evening before, I forgot to iron it. Ironing my uniform should not have been a problem except I could not find my iron. After a frantic search of my room, it dawned on me a friend had borrowed it. I really did not want to disturb my friend at this early morning hour, but necessity prevailed.

With my uniform pressed, I took one last glance at myself in the mirror. I actually felt like a nurse now and wondered why I even had to bother going to clinical that day. Then fear crept in again and the same worries from the night before came flooding back.

Well! When I finally got to the hospital, the RN assigned to my patient reported to me that my patient was elderly, didn't have any legs, was deaf, and didn't talk...this report did nothing to soothe my fears. However, I did manage to bathe her and change the bed linens without incident.

Giving her medications was a different story. I don't know whether she just didn't like me or maybe it was the pills, but she spit them out and they flew to the floor. Now I wondered what to do. Pick them up and administer them again? No, I reasoned I wouldn't want that done to me. I tried to remember if something like this had been discussed in class. Nothing came to mind. I went to the nurses' station and found my nurse and asked her what I should do. She instructed 'Just pick them up and try giving them to her again.' I wasn't sure I had heard her correctly, so I got my courage up and asked her what to do again...same response, 'Just pick them up and give them to her.' Even though my poor patient had dementia and wouldn't know the difference, I decided I better look for my instructor. Thankfully she informed me there was a very simple solution to my problem. She helped me pour out some new pills that we administered. This time my patient swallowed them without difficulty."

Melita concluded her story by informing me her first clinical day in the hospital taught her that sadly

"Not every nurse goes by what our books say." Then she added, "Good thing I was that patient's nurse that day!"

Like Melita, most of us encounter first "situation" jitters. Peaceful nights of sleep evade us as fear nudges images of our human frailties into our conscience. But we do have something great going for us. God has given us many, many promises to hold on to in situations where we need assurance and strength in times of crisis and in every ordinary day events. One in particular is found in Isaiah 41:13 & 14 God promises, "I am the Lord your God. I will strengthen you and hold your hand, so do not be afraid...Don't fear my children, I will help you..."

About those pills on the floor...not putting aside the sanitary issue, Melita did come up with a basic principle all of us should put into practice...don't do it if you wouldn't want it done to you.[1] Then at the end of the day just maybe the patient will appreciatively say, "Good thing you were my nurse today!"

Bonnie Hunt

Gifts Differing

"We really made a striking couple. Bill with his lopped sided grin and me hobbling around from my hysterectomy," mused Helen as she was telling me about her husband's parotid surgery and her recent hysterectomy. Helen had barely been discharged from the hospital when her husband had to go in for his surgery. Since I have a burden concerning the image of nursing, I asked Helen what had impressed her most from these two recent hospital experiences.

Grinning from ear to ear she recounted an incident that occurred early one morning as she was returning from the cafeteria with her breakfast tray to Bill's room. "This man from house keeping saw me hobbling down the ground floor hall with my hands full." "I see you need some help," he observed. "He proceeded to hold open the elevator door. I entered thinking that was nice of him to hold the door for me but his kindness did not end there. He also entered the elevator, pushed the button to my floor and went up the four flights with me, and then held the door open for me to exit and wished me a 'good day'." Helen continued, "I was expecting this gentleman from housekeeping to get off on this floor with me for a chore he had to do. But no, he helped me off and went back down to the ground floor to finish his chores there."

Helen insists that, people are frightened when they come to the hospital and are acutely aware how they are treated with each contact they make with hospital personnel. From the person in admissions to the person that cleans the room and even the person that discharges them. Helen concluded her comments with, "There were a few glitches, but the care was good and most everyone was pleasant, but the memory of the kindness of the man from housekeeping is what has stayed with me."

I didn't get the image of nursing I hoped for but I did get the picture of what a user- friendly institution should be.

The Apostle Paul tells us that we have been given "gifts differing."[1] "If you have received the gift of pastoral concern, then do that. Or, if you have the gift of teaching, then concentrate on that. If God has given you the gift to counsel and encourage others, do it. If you have the gift of administration, take your responsibilities seriously. If you've been given the capacity to show kindness and compassion, do it joyfully." Paul adds, "Be kind and courteous to one another as true brothers and sisters, honoring each other above yourselves. Don't be lazy; do your work enthusiastically, just as if the Lord Himself had employed you."

Bonnie Hunt

Having Done It for One of the Least

Cindi relates:

"Understaffed, underpaid, under appreciated! Understaffed, underpaid, under appreciated! Understaffed, under paid, under appreciated was a phase bouncing off my consciousness like a rubber ball bouncing up and down on the pavement. I was trying to cope with 30 severely mentally ill adult patients. These clients were incontinent, drooling, and hallucinating. Some had dried food on their clothes, some were in fetal position, and others were just milling about while some were quietly coloring with crayons in coloring books. I had medications to administer and blood glucose sticks with sliding scale insulin to draw up and administer. Then I needed to chart. But these people needed some physical care, and more importantly they needed 'tender loving care.' I was an 'agency' nurse with one assistant and to say the task was over whelming would be an understatement. Then on top of all this the assistant added a less than comforting thought by relating that recently one of the patients had 'stabbed' a nurse in the neck.

I complained to the supervisor that I did not have enough help, that the task was just too overwhelming, and I did not see how I was going to cope. Empathically she gave me a bit of advice I will never forget. She said, "Cindi, think of it this way, 'Inasmuch as you have done it unto one of the least of these, you have done it unto me.'"

The strangest thing happened. My tension slowly evaporated as 'Inasmuch as you have done it unto one of the least of these, you have done it unto me' kept resonating in my thoughts. I began to think just maybe I will be able to cope with this overwhelming situation.

Even so, my responsibilities were not without difficulties. Administering medications was very time consuming. I had to patiently coax some patients to open their clamped shut mouths as I attempted to give them their medicines; others I had to make sure they did not lose some of their medication in their drool. Still others shied away from me when they realized a needle "stick" was eminent. But surprisingly as the end of the shift approached, the assistant and I had time to get clean clothes on the patients that were incontinent and that had drool and dried food on them; others we tried to make comfortable in chairs or coached to watch some TV instead of milling aimlessly around. I even sat down and colored a picture with those that had been quietly coloring.

Now as I continue to do 'agency' nursing in a mental health setting the verses in Matthew 25:35-40 anchors me for the challenge. 'You have cared about others, which shows that you care about me. When others were thirsty, you gave them water. When they were hungry, you gave them food, and when they were without a place to live, you took them in. When they were sick, you visited and comforted them, and when they were in jail, you didn't forget them...What you did my caring for those who are thought to be unimportant was acknowledged by God as if you had done it for me.'"

Bonnie Hunt

The Return of Christmas Gifts

It was the first time that my new wife and I would not spend Christmas with our families.

We lived in Denver where I was attending nursing school and our families lived in Texas. My wife, Nettie, was a new RN and worked on the cardiac care unit at Porter Memorial Hospital. I worked as a technician in the Central Processing department of the hospital on weekends and evenings. Money was tight since I was in nursing school and could not work very much during each school semester. We had to budget for my tuition and books and were just beginning to pay on Nettie's school loans. Because of this, a trip to Texas was out of our reach not only because of the expense of the trip, but also due to the time lost at work. Missing our families, we felt sorry for ourselves, especially as our friends at school talked about their excitement anticipating going home and enjoying Christmas with their families.

Desiring to get out of our blue mood, we struggled with thinking of what we could do to make things better. Wanting to make a negative situation for us into making a positive one for others, we decided to volunteer to work Christmas Day, New Year's Day, and the week in between. This would allow someone else to get one of the holidays off to be home for Christmas. Instead of feeling blue while we worked over the holidays, we felt good that we could do a small act to allow someone else to enjoy a holiday with family.

Two years had passed since that Christmas. I was working as a registered nurse at a large county hospital in Austin, Texas, and was scheduled to work on Christmas Day on the 7-3 shift. Our first child, Brian, was five months old and this would be his first Christmas. It was probably more exciting for his parents' inner children than it was for him since he didn't even know Christmas was coming. I really did not want to miss the traditional waking up on Christmas morning and showing our baby the wonderments of opening presents in front of the Christmas tree all lit with twinkling lights. I didn't want to miss the Christmas candles and crisp invigorating smell of pine from the tree. In my mind, I imagined helping Brian open his first present and watch him laugh in glee as he saw a wonderful toy that he would play with for hours. (NOTE: If you are a parent reading this, you know right away that I was a new father. Babies are more interested in the wrapping paper, bows, and the box the toy comes in. The toy itself generates at least 60 seconds of interest with intense prompting from a parent.)

As a compromise, Nettie and I planned to have Christmas that evening after I got off work. It just wasn't the same, but I knew I needed to become accustomed to working holidays as a nurse. I went to work, again feeling sorry for myself, and sat in report with a glum look on my face.

"Something wrong?" the charge nurse asked as she looked at me across the table.

"Oh, nothing. I just miss spending Christmas morning with our new baby."

"Oh, that's right. This will be his first Christmas.", she said thoughtfully, "Well, maybe it will be a quiet day and you can get off on time."

"I hope so."

The shift began like any other shift on any other day. In spite of my disappointment at having to work, I greeted each patient with a "Merry Christmas" and a big smile. The routine of vital signs, medications, treatments, hygiene, and assessment went by swiftly that morning. Just before 11:00 a.m., the charge nurse called me into the office.

"Dave, how's your morning been?"

Inspiration PRN: Stories About Nurses

"It's been busy, but I am on schedule and I even have all of my charts up to date."

"That's great!" she said and then paused looking at me with a big smile on her face. "Dave, I have a Christmas present for you. I talked to the other nurses and we all agree. We want you to spend the rest of the day at home for your baby's first Christmas. I am sending you home and we will take care of your patients for the rest of the day." It turned out to be one of my favorite Christmases.

It was one of my favorite Christmases for two reasons. One reason being that I was able to spend it with my family and the other reason was that it was due to the people I worked with that made it possible. Many times you have heard that nurses do not take care of other nurses and that they "eat their young." Here was one example of nurses collaborating together to do an act of kindness. If everyone looked for opportunities to show kindness and caring, wouldn't the world be a better place?

David Gerstle

Singing Nurse Assistant

"Jesus loves me this I know, For the Bible tells me so; Little ones to Him belong, They are weak, but He is strong. Yes, Jesus loves me! Yes, Jesus loves me! Yes, Jesus loves me! The Bible tells me so."[1]

The words of this well-known song floated through the hallways of the hospital unit as the morning shift was well underway. The voice singing this melody was strong, clear, and full of conviction. Where was it coming from? I was quite curious so I began searching its source. Was it coming from a patient's room?

"Jesus loves me! He who died Heaven's gate to open wide"[1]

The second stanza seemed to be emanating from the second room on this hall.

"He will wash away my sin, Let His little child come in."

The patient's door was open. Inside was a new nurse assistant setting up the breakfast tray for the elderly female patient there.

"Yes Jesus loves me! Yes Jesus loves me! Yes Jesus loves me! The Bible tells me so."[1]

The nurse assistant with a beautiful smile on her face was singing to the patient at full volume, as the patient was a bit hard of hearing. The patient also had a beautiful smile on her face as she contentedly sat upright in her bed and listened to the concert.

It was a peaceful scene and I would have liked to stay there and enjoy the music also, but I had a full load of patients to care for and had to get to work. Maybe the nurse assistant would come and sing to one of my patients and I could hear some more music.

Inspiration PRN: Stories About Nurses

"There's a land that is fairer than day, And by faith we can see it afar: for the Father waits over the way, To prepare us a dwelling place there."[2]

The melody of this hymn was much closer now. In fact it was coming from one of my rooms. I really liked this song and I had to go listen more closely.

"In the sweet by and by, We shall meet on that beautiful shore."[2]

It was similar to the scene before. The singing nurse assistant was brushing the patient's hair as she sat in a chair. The patient looked quite content with her eyes closed as she listened to the comforting words of this hymn. All was peaceful.

I went about my duties as I listened to the singing. A short time later, I saw the nurse assistant walking down the hall. I wanted to meet the person behind the beautiful voice.

"Excuse me" I called after her.

Stopping and turning around, she looked my way to see who was speaking.

"I wanted to meet our singing nurse assistant. I'm David. I am one of the RNs who work on this floor."

"Hi, I'm Mary. I just started working here. Glad to meet you."

"I like your singing and I could tell the patients you were singing to were very pleased. That is really a nice thing for you to do."

Blushing a tiny bit, Mary explained to me that she believed God gave her a gift of singing and she wanted to share it with others. She took a nursing assistant position because she thought that ill patients would appreciate her singing the most.

"It's just a little thing to sing, but I feel like I am helping people feel better."

I replied, "If you saw the faces of those patients you were singing to you would know it was a big thing. They thought they were in heaven."

Mary thanked me for telling her that. I didn't sing to her (God didn't give me the gift of song), but a smile was on her face and she had a bounce in her walk as she headed down the hall.

We all have talents that God has given us. However, we don't always use them to benefit others around us. Perhaps it is because we underestimate the good our talents can provide or we don't think anyone would appreciate what we can do. Yet, what can be better use of our talents than to benefit others?

Many times we only consider abilities in the arts, music, or writing to be the only major talents. But, the ability to cook, garden, and build are notable talents. Abilities in interacting with people are also talents. Being sensitive to others' needs and doing something about them is a talent. Kindness and recognition of others' contributions and work are talents.

Over the years, I have seen many talented nurses share their talents. What can you do with your talents to make another's life a bit brighter? How about bringing flowers grown in your garden for patients to enjoy? Are you a poet? Share your poems with your patients. Sharing artwork is another gift. The gift of listening is a precious talent. Take some time out of your hectic shift and listen to a patient. This is a precious gift not often given. The patient will never forget you for giving this time. What about humor? If you have a good sense of humor, share this with your patients and co-workers. Seeing the funnier side of otherwise serious situations can be a real stress buster; you must be careful not to offend or be insensitive, but it does wonders for those involved. Being funny is a real talent and does wonders for those lacking in endorphins.

Can you cook, bake, or grow vegetables? A loaf of bread or a batch of chocolate chip cookies is highly prized by those who work with you. Bringing a tasty dish for potlucks at work is another means to share your cooking talent.

Recognizing and affirming others is another talent to share. Take time to tell another co-worker or boss that you appreciate them and why. Think of a specific thing that you appreciate and tell them. A fellow nurse will appreciate hearing something like "I am always glad when we work together because I know we will help each other. A boss would always welcome someone saying, "I appreciate you always trying to get us enough staff." It is especially important to tell service personnel such as housekeepers, technicians, and clerks how much you appreciate them. You will be amazed how good this will make them feel.

We may not all be able to sing like Mary, but we all have God-given talents that can be a benefit to others and perhaps give a picture of God and His love for us.

"This little light of mine, I'm going to let it shine. Let it shine, Let it shine."[3]

"Let you light so shine before men, that they may see your good works and glorify your Father in heaven."[4]

David Gerstle

Inspiration PRN: Stories About Nurses

SPIRITUAL LIFE— FIRST THINGS FIRST

A Bedpan by Any Other Name...

It was only our second clinical lab in the hospital as spanking brand new student nurses. We had practiced in the skills lab at the school in preparation for wielding our newly learned skills on real patients. Our first day in the hospital was spent taking vital signs and talking to our patients. We were assigned in pairs to one patient. This was more for our comfort and perhaps the patient's safety in that maybe two student nurses together would not decide to do something dangerous to the patient.

Having survived the first lab, our second lab was designed to give a bedbath to a patient. All of us had practiced this art on each other (in bathing suits of course and not in mixed company) in skills lab. Now, our clinical instructor pronounced we were indeed ready to bathe the world! Well, our assigned patient anyway. This time it was one-on-one and not in pairs.

Nursing students take a lot more time to complete a task such as a bedbath. Those of us who finished first were congregating around the nurses' station afterwards awaiting our instructor's acknowledgment that we had indeed performed this momentous nursing duty.

"How did your bedbath go?" one of my student peers asked me.

"Well, no one got hurt. May even had cleaned off some dirt," I jokingly replied. "How was yours?" I asked.

"About the same, the patient and I both survived."

While we were exchanging comments about giving baths, Karen, one of our other peers walks up to us wiping down a gleaming silver metal bedpan. She has a big grin on her face and proudly announces to us, "Guess what, guys? I have just completed my first bedbath!"

Inspiration PRN: Stories About Nurses

"From that?" I asked, nodding to the bedpan.

"Well, sure, what's wrong with that?" Karen asked with a confused look on her face.

"Do you think that is a bath basin?" my other buddy asks.

It was at this moment that lightening hit Karen's brain with the realization that she just bathed her first patient out of a bedpan.

"OH NO!" Karen exclaimed. "I can't believe I did that." She was torn between laughing and crying. Her face was turning a brilliant crimson color as she clutched the now very shiny bedpan as she was still nervously polishing it with a towel.

"What am I going to do?" she cried out.

"You may want to consider a re-do on that bath you just gave," I quickly suggested.

My other buddy adds, "You may want to take that bedpan back to your patient's room. Here comes our instructor."

Karen may not have been able to tell the difference between a bedpan and a bath basin, but she knew to avoid a potentially fatal and humiliating encounter with our no-nonsense teacher. Needless to say, the patient got another bath (from a basin) by Karen since she felt rather bad about the situation. She told the patient she wanted to get her extra clean and she never told her she had first received a bedpan bath (although I am not sure how the patient didn't notice the pan) and we never told the instructor what catastrophe had lurked behind the patient's door.

Maybe you have never given a bath out of a bedpan, but have you ever tried to make yourself spiritually clean by your own goodness? Perhaps you have tried to be righteous by virtue of doing your own good works. Maybe you have desired to work out your own salvation. Yet, isn't this just like trying to get clean by bathing out of a bedpan. It may look clean when you use it, but we all know where it has been.

The only way to be spiritually clean is by accepting Jesus Christ as your personal Savior. By accepting His sacrifice on the cross is the only way to have His Cleanliness in our lives. By accepting Him, His good works are accounted to us. Have you bathed in His Righteousness to become spiritually clean? Have you been washed by the Holy Spirit?

"Not by works of righteousness which we have done, but according to his mercy he saved us, by the washing of regeneration, and renewing of the Holy Ghost; which He shed on us abundantly through Jesus Christ our Saviour."[1]

David Gerstle

Windy Wake-Up Call

    The hospital had been very busy the past few weeks. The census was high and the staff was stretched to the limit. It was the beginning of summer and therefore the nursing staff was ready for long overdue and well-deserved vacations. Since hospitals are open 365 days a year, vacations had to be staggered in order to provide safe staffing. This shift was the last one for me before starting my vacation. I had worked the 3 p.m.-11 p.m. shift last night and was now finishing up the 7 a.m.-3 p.m. shift today. Having only slept a few hours, I was tired, but the thought of vacation spurred me on. Finally the last chart was signed off and shift report given, I was off for two weeks with the family to vacation in Florida and visit Mickey Mouse.

    The summer heat beat down on me as I walked to my truck in the parking lot. Opening the truck door released even more heat into the sweltering atmosphere. It was an old truck with a non-functioning air conditioner, so I surrendered myself to its hot cauldron of a cab for the 45-minute drive home. With the windows rolled down and the fan going full blast, I pulled out onto the highway. As the Texas scenery of pastures and cows flew by, I thought of beaches and the Magic Kingdom. Suddenly, I felt the truck being pushed to one side of the road and gripped the steering wheel making my knuckles turn white! Now fully alert, I checked the rear and side mirrors. There were no other vehicles near me so no one had hit me. It could have been a gust, but strangely there was no sign of any wind. None of the trees or shrubs was being blown about, even though the wind seemed to have pushed my truck around. There was no dust swirling from the dry fields; no litter blowing across the road.

Was I imagining things? Maybe I startled myself falling asleep at the wheel and woke up just in time to keep my truck on the road. Perhaps it could be rationalized away and be interpreted as a coincidental and fortunate set of events. On the other hand, maybe there wasn't any typical wind blowing that day. Maybe God sent a windy wake-up call just in time and just enough to keep me from harm. Whatever it was, it certainly worked as I was no longer sleepy and arrived home safe and ready for a vacation.

Sometimes our spiritual life becomes too comfortable and we become inattentive to our relationship with God. We become "sleepy" and just go through the motions as we travel down life's road, growing less alert and more complacent on our journey. Crisis, results of poor choices, and temptations can either push us further into our spiritual somnolence or jerk us awake. God, at these times, sends His Spirit for us to call on Him for help and strength. For some, He can speak through a gentle breeze, for others (like me!), He must roar as a mighty wind. May God keep you alert spiritually as you travel down life's road.

"Most assuredly, I say to you, unless one is born of water and the Spirit, he cannot enter the kingdom of God. That which is born of the flesh is flesh, and that which is born of the Spirit is spirit. Do not marvel that I said to you, 'You must be born again'. The wind blows where it wishes, and you hear the sound of it, but cannot tell where it comes from and where it goes. So is everyone who is born of the Spirit."[1]

David Gerstle

Living Water

A ramshackle shack of a house on the side of a mountain was the home of an elderly husband and wife, Raymond and Della Duda. It didn't seem to matter to them that the house was poorly insulated against the harsh elements and that they did not have indoor pluming. It didn't seem to matter that the foam rubber in their couch cushions was crumbling under faded threadbare upholstery. It didn't seem to matter that their kitchen table and chairs wobbled on the uneven wood planks that served as a floor. It didn't seem to matter that wooden crates used as kitchen cupboard was as bare as "old mother Hubbard's cupboard." They had each other and "dog."

Raymond did the best he could to care for Della after she fell and broke her hip. But Raymond did not know that continuous pressure on soft tissues between bony prominences compresses capillaries and occludes blood flow causing damage to the underlying tissue. The inevitable happened. A pressure ulcer developed on the sacrum. Now it became necessary for a community health nurse to make daily trips through the mud to the little shack. Kathy was assigned this task. It was during the first visit that a special bond developed between nurse and this frail elderly couple. Kathy looked forward to her daily visits and providing ulcer care. However, after a few weeks it became evident that Della's care was too much for Raymond. So arrangements were made for Della to be placed in a long-term health care facility.

Concerned over having to separate this devoted couple, Kathy made a visit to the health care facility expecting to find a sad and homesick Della. Sparkling eyes and a grin from ear to ear greeted Kathy as she entered Della's room. "How are you doing?" asked Kathy.

Inspiration PRN: Stories About Nurses

"Guess what?" Della enthused. "I get corn bread that has butter on it every day and they put me in this big tub where water comes right out of the wall and you can get water anytime you want by turning a knob." Kathy related, "Della's enthusiasm made her sound as if she was describing the 'Hilton'."

It is difficult to believe in this age of "hi tech" that one would not be aware that water "comes right out of the wall" and is very accessible by just "turning a knob." However, I wonder how many of us are like Della, not aware that "living" water is plentiful and always available any time we need it by just turning the knob of prayer. "Living" water is special. "Once you drink it you will never be thirsty again. It will constantly bubble up inside of you like a fresh mountain spring, furnishing eternal life."[1] If we drink this living water then we might be just like Della, eyes sparkling and a grin from ear to ear. And shouldn't we share with others just like Della did with Kathy that "living" water is plentiful and always available just by turning the knob of prayer?

Postscript:

On another visit Della shared with Kathy her worries. "Raymond is not doing so good and he refuses to go see a doctor." It was a sheriff that noticed he had not seen Raymond for a few days and went out to check on him. Raymond was dead and lying on the floor. "Dog" was lying on top of him growling and showing his teeth daring anyone to come near his master. Della spent her remaining days, sad but content, where water came out of the wall and she could get water anytime she wanted just by turning a knob.

Bonnie Hunt

Good Medicine

"Laughter is the sun that drives winter from the human face," is a favorite quote of mine by Victor Hugo. Some might surmise there is little to laugh about when providing nursing care for the sick and suffering...wrong! Sometimes it is those incidents that make us smile that keep us from buckling under the stress.

It seems a travesty to me now, but in the olden days parents were only allowed to visit their hospitalized child on Tuesday and Thursday afternoons for an hour. So, five-year-old Johnny was left alone in his hospital crib the evening prior to his surgery for strabismus. A charming little rascal, he was and not the least bit shy. "Chatter box" doesn't do him justice but will have to suffice for the lack of a better adjective.

Unfortunately, it was one of those shifts that one hopes is not repeated very often. Nurses running to and fro past Johnny's room would entice him to call out, "Nurse! Nurse!" Come in here and play with me." Getting no response for a playmate he would then call out "I need you nurse." When one of us would go into his room to see what he wanted he would point to a toy he had thrown out of his bed or say he wanted a sip of water or go "umm, I think I need some medicine."

By the end of the shift he was still awake but had settled down some. Making my last rounds for the evening I was able to take a few minutes to confront this little charmer and wondered how he was going to react when he came back from surgery the next day with both eyes bandaged.

As soon as I arrived for my shift the next day I found Johnny sitting somewhat subdued in his crib tugging at the bandages covering both his eyes. "Oh! Johnny don't touch your bandages," I exclaimed. "You will undo all the work the doctor has done." Turning in the direction of my voice he replied, "Nurse, I won't touch these bandages if you will only turn on the lights and pull up the shades." I don't think I wiped that smile off my face for days.

However, there are too many shifts that leave nurses humorless and burned out. So it is these unexpected humorous events that buoy us up...even if we have to laugh at our selves. Like the time a patient rang his call light and the nurse answered, "May I help you?"

"Can you come down here?"

"I'll be there in a minute."

"Is that a real minute or a nurse's minute?"

Mary, a nursing assistant tells about checking on a patient that was due to go for a test and was NPO. The patient's granddaughter (a woman in her 30's) was sitting at her bedside. The granddaughter asked if it was O.K. to wipe her grandmother's head with a damp washcloth. Mary told her that it was fine and the granddaughter replied, "I know I can't put it by her mouth." Confused, Mary asked her "why?" Her answer: "The sign on the door says nothing by mouth."

"Working as a certified nurse assistant in a long term health care facility is not easy but rewarding work," confided Kelly now a nursing student. "However there were incidences that made my work enjoyable. I still get a chuckle over the time I walked into a female residents room to get her up for the afternoon. As I was getting ready to get her up, I realized I didn't have an adult brief, which she needed. I explained 'I'll be right back, I need to get a diaper.'" As I was leaving the room she called out "Honey, bring me one too."

Those that work with pediatric patients probably could fill a book with laughter. An ER nurse tells about a precocious four year old that was brought to the ER with a chief complaint of cough and difficulty breathing. She kept up a nonstop conversation while the nurse was trying to assess her heart rate and lung sounds. Finally the nurse said, "Shhh, I have to see if Barney is in there." The child looked up and calmly stated, "I have Jesus in my heart. Barney is on my underwear."

Then there was Mark...born with one ventricle. He spent much of his childhood in and out of hospitals. This time he was in with fluid overload. He was sneaking so many drinks they had to lock his bathroom door. He protested, but finally settled down to play. He decided to be artistic and set up his paper and paints. It seemed innocent, until he asked to "fill this cup with water for my paints. Very, very cold water, please."

One of my favorite chuckling events occurred while Art Linkletter was touring a nursing home. He approached a sweet white-haired lady in a wheel chair, shook her hand and said, "Do you know who I am?" "No," she replies, "But if you go to the nurse's station they'll tell you who you are."

Humor is a basic human need. Make the humor in your work a health issue. It's a Biblical principle. "A merry heart is good medicine, but a broken spirit dries out the bones."[1]

Bonnie Hunt

The Healing Word

The neurology unit sprung to life as usual right at change of shift in the morning. Surgical patients needed to be ready when the OR department called for them. Vital signs and assessments had to be completed and preoperative medications given. Last-minute final review of the patients' charts to check for all the proper consents, signatures, and other necessary documents added to the controlled chaos of a busy hospital nursing unit.

This morning the unit clerk was busy transcribing physician orders, scheduling labwork and other tests for the early morning admissions. When one of the phones rung at the desk, I answered it, "Unit 300, this is Gerstle, RN."

"Hi Dave, this is Debbie in OR. Go ahead and preop Mrs. Clark in room 330. We will be there in about 15 minutes." "OK, Deb, consider it done." I said to the OR clerk.

Mrs. Clark had been assigned to me that day so I drew up the preoperative medications after checking the chart and medication record. I knew the Clark's well as I had taken care of Mr. Clark when he had back surgery a few months before. He had worked for years in a railroad yard in the small town of Cleburne, Texas, and had retired there still living in the same house he had bought when they were newlyweds 40 years before. The couple was growing old together and completely devoted to each other.

Mrs. Clark had been admitted to the hospital for surgery after a brain tumor had been discovered by CT scan. Her doctors felt confident that it could be successfully removed, however, the surgeon had warned the patient there was a risk the surgery could cause

Inspiration PRN: Stories About Nurses

some neurological loss or the tumor may be found inoperable. Mrs. Clark was a sincere Christian and told the surgeon that she had faith God would guide his hands during the operation and allow her to be healed.

Her hospital room door was partly open as I approached her room with the medications. As I peered inside, I saw Mrs. Clark lying in bed with an opened Bible resting on her forehead. Mr. Clark was asleep in a chair next to the window. As I knocked lightly on the door, I greeted the patient with a "Good Morning," chuckling as I did so. Mrs. Clark opened her eyes and removed the Bible from her head.

"Good morning, Doctor Dave*. Good to see you, but why are you laughing?"

"Well," I drawled, "You have a Bible on your head and it, well, it tickled my funny bone." I felt a bit sheepish now; I hadn't laughed out loud, I just couldn't quite suppress my amusement, as an experienced registered nurse should be capable to do.

"Son, where is your faith? Don't you know what the Bible says about the power of God's Word? Don't you know His Word heals?"

Uh, oh, now I know I really should not have laughed. About this time, Mr. Clark awakens, listening to the one-sided conversation.

"Hey, it's Dr. Dave, Good morning!"

I greeted him as Mrs. Clark continued to tell me I needed to shore up my faith in no uncertain terms.

Mrs. Clark was about 65 years old and a confident strong woman with conviction in her unwavering faith in God. She wasn't going to let an opportunity to pass to speak of her faith. She also wasn't going to let anyone underestimate her Lord's abilities either.

"Boy, you done it now. Mama don't like it if she thinks your faith is weak. We gonna have "church" right

---

* I explained to them many times that I was a registered nurse, but the Clarks insisted on calling me Dr. Dave.

here and now." Mr. Clark is laughing while he is telling me this.

I'm now really feeling embarrassed, not to mention anxious since I also needed to preop the woman. Mrs. Clark continues, "The Bible says in Psalms that He sent His Word and healed them. My head needs healing so that's where the Word is going." And with that, she replaced her Bible on her head.

I humbly apologized to Mrs. Clark for laughing when I knocked on the door.

"No need to apologize to me, but you best be praying to God and know that He can heal us through His Word."

And we did pray, the Clarks and I. We prayed for a successful surgery and healing and, yes, for more faith for me. The preoperative medications were given and the OR orderly wheeled her away on a gurney. Despite hospital regulations, Mrs. Clark took her Bible with her, resting comfortably on her head.

Faith in God is often strongest in its simplest form. We tend to overanalyze the prospects of whether God will answer our prayers and thus rationalize our faith away. Simple faith is taking God at His word and allowing Him to guide our lives, always depending on Him. David in Psalms 30:2 showed his faith when he wrote, "O Lord my God, I cried out to You and You have healed me." Perhaps Mrs. Clark's belief in literally applying God's word to her head is questionable but her faith in God was beyond question. Her faith was simple, yet strong.

"He sent His word and healed them, and delivered them from their destructions."[1]

Post Script: Mrs. Clark's surgery was successful and she was completely healed. I would see them occasionally at the grocery store after she recovered. They still called me Dr. Dave.

David Gerstle

Christmas Code Blue

We were hoping for a nice slow Christmas shift in the hospital that evening. I was a nursing student in my junior year and worked in the Central Processing Department at a large metropolitan hospital in Colorado. Christmas Day dawned clear and cold. From our apartment window, Nettie, my new bride, and I could see the Rockies covered in snow. My wife was a brand new RN who worked in the cardiac unit at the hospital. We both worked the 3-11 shift. Not having enough money to return home to Texas for Christmas with the family, we both volunteered to work the holidays. Don, who was also a nursing student, and his wife Sharon were also staying for the holidays, too. Don worked with me in the Central Processing department at the hospital and his wife worked at a local bank.

Nettie, Don, and I were scheduled to work the 3-11 shift at the hospital. We had decided to share Christmas dinner before going to work. The meal was a virtual feast with all the trimmings: mashed potatoes, green bean casserole, pies, cakes, and of course the traditional Adventist facsimile turkey and dressing. Enjoying the meal so much, we had agreed to save dessert for a late night snack after work. With great effort, the three of us who had to work this evening forced ourselves from the table. We waddled down the stairs from Don and Sharon's upstairs apartment. The apartments where we lived were within walking distance to the hospital; so we began our post-feast journey to work. As we stepped onto the sidewalk to the hospital, Don turned around to wave goodbye to his wife who was watching us from their apartment window. Tears moistened her cheeks as she anticipated being alone that evening. Nettie and I turned around and waved also, feeling a little sad for her and Don and a little sad for ourselves having to work. But then, we all realized that the patients in the hospital were away from their homes and ill or injured. This broke down our "feeling sorry for ourselves" moment and motivated us along the sidewalk.

Nettie headed upstairs to the cardiac unit and Don and I headed downstairs into the bowels of the hospital where Central Processing was located. Changing into scrubs, Don and I entered the department and clocked in. Part of the responsibilities of the technicians was to respond to Code Blues that were called during the shift. We carried to the cardiopulmonary emergency additional supplies and equipment and handed what was needed to the code team. We also ran any blood gases to the Lab for analysis and helped where needed. This provided great experiences for nursing students, however, tonight, Christmas night, I hoped we would not have any codes. It was my turn to respond to any codes called, so the first task at hand was to check the Code Blue supply cart that we took with us. All was in order, so it was time to settle into the routine of wrapping surgical packs and instruments. Don was working the steam sterilizers and Joan, the head technician, was working the gas sterilizers and, of course, supervising Don and me. That was in itself a full time job.

The phone was quiet this evening and we were thankful for the reprieve from a usually hectic shift. We talked as we worked, reminiscing over past Christmases and what our plans were for the rest of the holiday week. Then our quiet reverie came to a screeching halt when the inevitable happened.

"Code Blue CCU," the PA system crackled into life.

"Code Blue, CCU," the operator on the PA repeated.

"Code Blue, CCU" intoned the third time.

Springing into action, I put on my lab coat over my scrubs. Joan grabbed the cart and pushed it to me as I raced out of the door and down the hall to the elevators.

Inspiration PRN: Stories About Nurses

A family with three little children were in the hall as I rushed toward them. The mother grabbed her children as they giggled watching me in my scrubs and surgical cap push the cart down the corridor.

"Excuse me." I said as I rushed by.

The CCU was on the second floor and on the other side of the hospital. As I entered the doors of the unit, I quickly spotted where the code was in full progress. Nurses, respiratory therapists, supervisors, and the cardiologist were all intensely performing their duties to save the patient's life. One nurse was performing chest compressions as another was pushing IV cardiac medications. A respiratory therapist was "bagging" the patient through an endotracheal tube. The cardiologist was yelling out orders for medications and blood gases.

In the center of the code lay the patient; pale and to all appearances lifeless. I found out later that he was a devoted 35 year-old husband and father of a son, a boy in elementary school. He had suffered a myocardial infarction and was brought in by ambulance on Christmas Eve. He had suffered one other heart attack prior to this one during the day and survived. It was around seven in the evening and this time it did not look good for him. The CCU nursing staff was experienced veterans who were on the top of their field. The cardiologist this evening was also well experienced and was the chief of the cardiology department. If there was a chance to save this patient, this team could do it.

As the team worked on the patient, demands on me increased.

"Dave, grab me another IV pump!"

"Dave, I need some primary IV tubing."

"Dave, run this blood gas to the lab."

As I returned from the lab with the blood gas results, no further progress had been made in the code. CPR was being vigorously administered but without results. The patient remained pale and motionless. At this moment, the patient's wife rushed into the CCU and sees the code team trying to resuscitate her husband. I will never forget seeing on her face the look of horror and at the same time a look of determination to save her husband's life. Perhaps it was my mind's own interpretation, but her expression seemed to say to her husband:

"I will trade my life for yours so that you will live."

She broke into a run toward her husband as if to save him. I was the only person between her and where the code was taking place. As an inexperienced nursing student I did not know what to do. Should I grab her? Should I do nothing? Should I get in front of her? I didn't know and I didn't have much time to decide as she was quickly coming toward me. Not a moment too soon, the hospital chaplain appears at her side, takes her by the arm, and takes her to the family counseling room. I was never more glad to see a hospital chaplain in my life.

As the code continued, it was soon evident that this 35-year-old man would not live. The most modern knowledge, medications, and technology were done to no avail. Having resigned to this horrible outcome, the cardiologist "called" the code to a stop. These veteran healthcare professionals had participated in many codes and had learned to cope with the stress of them. Yet, it seemed that this code was different for them. Perhaps it was because it was Christmas or the young age of the patient, as the team was strongly affected. The nurse giving cardiac compressions would not stop; she continued until the physician put his arms around her and took her hands off of the patient's chest. She began to sob, as this had been her patient. The charge nurse mercifully instructed her to take a moment in the break room. The respiratory therapist placed his head in his hands and leaned against the wall, slowly sitting on the floor. The cardiologist just stood at the bedside, rubbing his eyes with one hand as he held his glasses with the other. As the other nurse and charge nurse began postmortem care, both had tears in their eyes. I helped pick up the discarded supplies and their packaging left in the aftermath. No one talked as we went about our duties. Slowly the team recovered and dispersed to each of our respective areas, as there were many more patients who needed care in the hospital. No more time for crying or being upset until the shift was over. We all had to cope with what Christmas had brought.

Yet through the rest of the shift, I reflected on the events of that evening. I wondered what the chaplain had said to the wife when he took her to the counseling room. I pondered how he and the cardiologist told the patient's wife that her husband did not survive. I also wondered how this wife and mother told her children that their father had died. I wondered how the nurses cared for the wife as she said goodbye to her deceased husband in the CCU.

I could not get out of my mind the look of the patient's wife when she saw her husband during the code. You could see the horror of the realization she had that her husband was dying and she would not see him again on this earth. You could tell that she deeply loved him and would have done anything, even give up her life, to save him if it was in her power to do so.

The loss of this young husband and father and the emotions that followed on this Christmas Day were all due to a "bad heart." Sometimes only a heart transplant can prevent death.

Spiritual death assuredly occurs without a "spiritual" heart transplant. Christmas is a special day when we celebrate the birth of the One who can give us a new heart. Our Lord and Savior gave up His life so that we may live. He transplants His character and thus gives each of us a good heart to replace our one. In order to keep His good heart in our lives, we must stay on life support with God. It is His goodness alone that saves

Inspiration PRN: Stories About Nurses

and it is His will that we live eternally with Him. Through Jesus Christ's birth and death, this patient and his wife can be reunited again when He returns.

As nurses we must share this hope with our patients as opportunities present themselves. It is a comfort only known to those who believe in the saving grace of our Lord's sacrifice. It is a hope that can only be experienced with a new heart from God.

"A new heart also will I give you, and a new spirit will I put within you: and I will take away the stony heart out of your flesh, and I will give you a heart of flesh."[1]

David Gerstle

Dismayed

"You cannot imagine the shock it is for patients and family to hear the doctor say 'you have cancer'", commented Helen an oncology nurse. "I am sure they must feel like the television commercial that says when you hear you have cancer it is like being dropped off a boat, left alone and you don't know how to swim. It is a particular blow when the patient has had no health problems and "something" showed up during a routine physical. This was the case with Mr. Haynes." Helen continued, "It was routine laboratory test that an elevated protein was noted which ultimately lead to a diagnosis of multiple myeloma. Shock is probably an understatement for what Mr. Haynes and his wife felt when the doctor told them Mr. Haynes's diagnosis. He had just retired and had been in good health with plans for travel and building a winter home in Florida."

Helen carefully and patiently explained what Mr. Haynes was to expect from his first chemotherapy treatment. The first "round" of chemotherapy was an oral dose that he was to take for six months and then have follow up laboratory tests. The Haynes postponed their plans and faithfully carried out the prescribed treatment. After six months, laboratory tests revealed protein levels within normal range. So, it was off to Florida and a good time. Returning back home for more followup laboratory tests, the results were disappointing, the protein levels were elevated again.

"Now we are going to have a more aggressive chemotherapy treatment. This 'round' of chemotherapy will be with intravenous drugs. They will cause you to be ill with nausea, vomiting, dizziness and your hair will fall out," warned Helen.

As Helen continued with her instructions she silently wondered how many patients over the years she had given these very same instructions and how very ill her patients had become with these particular drugs.

"Even though I knew this precious couple had a strong faith and a faithful pray life, I felt a particular sadness for what theses drugs were going to put them though," related Helen.

During the treatment Helen called to check on Mr. Haynes. When Helen asked to speak to Mr. Haynes, Mrs. Haynes said he was out painting the house. Astonished Helen inquired, "Is he nauseated? "No-oo" was the reply. "Well if he is dizzy, he should not be on a ladder," continued Helen. "Well he is not dizzy...he is not sick and the house needs painting," responded Mrs. Haynes. Helen said her disbelief was so compelling she made several more calls inquiring about Mr. Haynes's condition. Same response, no nausea, no vomiting, no dizziness and no hair falling out. "I was beginning to feel like I was having a "Jonah experience" and that the Haynes' would view me as a false prophet because my warnings did not materialize." lamented Helen. "The side efforts never did materialized and it left me completely dismayed."

After tests revealed Mr. Haynes' protein levels had decreased, the Haynes's referred to the experience as "positive faith." "Prayer and a positive attitude can go along way," insists Mrs. Haynes. "The Lord will go with you. He will not forsake you. Fear not, neither be dismayed."[1]

With the exception of the drug prednisone, Mr. Haynes rarely experienced a side effect during his ten years of treatment for multiple myeloma. As for Helen, Isaiah 55:8 and 9 took on new meaning. "The Lord says, 'My thoughts are not your thoughts, neither are my ways your ways. The heavens are higher than the earth, so are my thoughts higher than your thoughts and my ways higher than your ways."

Bonnie Hunt

Unusual? Maybe Not

    They were mingling in the lobby of the nursing building, their smiles and casual chatter masking the anxiety of the upcoming exam. It had been a tough semester and this exam was critical for several of their classmates. Graduation was just weeks away. A few minutes before 9:00 a.m. when the exam was to begin, the students started to file into the student lounge and invited me to join them. They gathered around in a close circle while Jenn opened her Bible and claimed several promises. "For I know the plans I have for you. Plans to prosper and not harm you, to give you a future and a hope."[1] "Don't be afraid for I am with you...I will uphold you with my victorious right hand."[2] Before bowing their heads to pray, Jenn commented, "We need to especially pray for Janice and Barbara since passing this test is so critical for them." Then we all bowed our heads and Jenn offered a prayer reminding God of his promises and asked for a special portion of wisdom to be given to the two students that were in jeopardy.

    "Well, I certainly am touched and impressed!" I commented as we left the lounge. "Oh! We have done this before every test since we began nursing with EVERY classmate participating," enthused Shannon.

    I was curious as to how the class was going to respond when I found out that the two students that they made a special petition for had failed the exam. They seemed a little more anxious but optimistic the next day as they gathered for the final exam. As these students had done all through their nursing education, they gathered in the lounge for claiming promises and prayer and again made a special request for the two classmates.

Inspiration PRN: Stories About Nurses

Later that day I saw the students with glorious smiles and thumbs up letting me know ALL had passed. With much encouragement and study support from their classmates, the two students that were struggling had made a high enough score on the final to give them a passing grade. These students' faith never wavered for they felt their devotion to claiming promises and prayer would pay off. And it did!

I mused to myself, this class was unusual because it was smaller than most nursing classes, but was comforted to think that at least some young people are still seeking God's guidance for their lives.

The notion that this graduating class was unusual was pleasantly shattered the next day as I passed the student lounge and heard the sweet melody of "Near-er, still near-er, close to Thy heart, Draw me, my Sav-iour, so precious Thou art; Fold me, O fold me close to Thy breast, Shelt-er me safe in that hav-en of rest,..." wafting through the air. Here was another class of nursing students in the lounge preparing for an upcoming exam. Their custom was to pick out a favorite hymn, sing, pray and then give each other encouraging hugs as part of their preparation for each exam.

Hooray for our future nurses!

Bonnie Hunt

Promises

It had been an intense study session. Since "failing" the last test, the soon to be taken test would be a determining link to Eva's progression in the nursing fundamentals class. A career in nursing was a life long dream for Eva, and the thought of "failing out" was more then she could bear. Turning to me with pleading eyes, Eva explained, "I get so nervous when I take these tests," and then asked, "What do you do about 'test anxiety'? I try to read all of the assignments and study the notes, but when I get to the test I begin to feel so anxious, that when I look at the choice of answers for the question they ALL look right." We had already gone over some test taking techniques like cover up the options, make sure you know what the question is asking, try to answer the question first and then look at the options one at a time. We also had talked about the importance of prayer. Now I sensed she needed more encouragement.

I have a folder that contains some printed pearlized sheets of paper with an attractive border that is titled "*God's Wonderful Promises to Claim for NCLEX.*" I pulled one of these sheets from the folder and gave it to Eva explaining that here were some promises that we give to encourage the students preparing for the National Council Licensure Exam (NCLEX). As she glanced over the promises she looked at me with the most engaging smile and exclaimed, "We need these now! Don't wait until NCLEX time to give them to us." I suggested she look them over and memorize one that would be helpful to her. I also told her about a student who wrote her memorized promise at the top of the sheet of paper she used to cover up her answers while she was reading the questions. And when she felt anxiety creeping in, she

Inspiration PRN: Stories About Nurses

would stop and read the promise and it calmed her down.

A few days later Eva was in my office with another student, Melinda, who was agonizing over her test anxiety. I produced another "promise" sheet. e sat around for a few minutes looking over the promises with Melinda trying to decide which promise would comfort her most. Finally Eva broke the silence, "That very first promise on the sheet gives me tremendous encouragement and is my favorite...'For I know the plans I have for you. Plans to prosper and not harm you...to give you a future and a hope'."[1] Then Eva related to Melinda how she wrote that promise down as soon as she started her last test. When she felt anxious, she would stop for a moment and read it. Eva continued, "Even though I always pray for wisdom before each test, claiming this promise during the test kept me focused on God being with me all through the test." Flashing that irresistible smile of hers, Eva continued, "I passed the test and plan to keep this practice with all my tests. Now I have confidence that God is giving me a 'future and a hope'."

"Give all your worries and cares to God, for He cares about what happens to you."[2]

Claiming His wonderful promises is a great way to give your anxieties, fears and worries to God. Try one today!

Bonnie Hunt

NEVER GIVE UP

Never Give Up!

Jim was a promising football star for the local high school. It was his senior year and the college scouts were watching this talented halfback. A scholarship to a top school could have been a reality. That is, until the car wreck.

One Saturday evening, Jim and a football buddy decided to go out to eat and then cruise along the "strip." It was a popular activity for the teenagers in town. Leaving the restaurant, the boys pulled out into the busy Saturday traffic and entered the freeway. Suddenly, a car flew past them in the next lane. It was swerving back and forth. Without warning, the car veered in front of them. Unable to stop in time, there was a tremendous crash as the two cars collided into each other. Jim and the rest of the boys were thrown about as the cars finally came to a grinding stop. An eerie silence fell over this gruesome scene of twisted metal and broken bodies. Motorists stopped and gave assistance until the ambulances and police arrived bringing with them the reality of this serious accident. The other boy in Jim's car was killed. The driver of the other car was also killed. Jim survived, but was in critical condition, having sustained a serious head injury and other trauma from the impact.

I met Jim a month or so after he was transferred from the ICU to the neurology unit at the hospital where I worked. He had severe neurological deficits. He could not yet walk or speak. He had limited use of his arms and required total assistance.

One skill Jim had acquired was to blink his eyes once for "yes" and twice for "no." All communication with him was dependent on this skill. Any chance he would improve seemed to also be dependent on it as well.

Jim's daily routine consisted of physical therapy, hygiene, and visits from his family. His mother and father were determined that Jim would recover. They ensured that all staff working with their son displayed a positive and hopeful attitude.

The first day I was assigned to Jim as his nurse, I approached him as I did all patients on the neurology unit. I greeted him, making sure I made eye contact with him. I spoke to him as if he could understand everything I said. As I greeted his mother next, she thanked me for speaking directly to her son.

"You know, some hospital staff won't talk directly to Jim. But, I think it is important if he is ever going to get better."

"I agree, the more stimulation he gets, the better."

She showed me all of the things in his room that provided positive stimulation. There were cards from his high school friends and pictures of him in his football uniform. His trophies were also displayed in the room. His parents brought in bright colorful posters and stuffed animals.

Throughout the day, his mother would talk to Jim and brush his hair or give him range of motion exercises. She would tell him what was going on with the rest of the family and what they were all going to do when he was better. It seemed so optimistic to expect Jim to progress much beyond where he was now. He couldn't even talk or make purposeful movement. The most he could do was sit up with full assistance and then had to be propped with pillows and strapped in his chair. In spite of this, his mother saw her son walking and talking again.

Was this a blind cruel faith in the impossible? Most experts in the field might think that the best hoped for would be that Jim could progress to needing only moderate levels of assistance in his activities of daily living. No one would expect him to continue school or work. However, a mother and father's faith was strong.

A few months later Jim transferred to a rehabilitation hospital. His parents came by and gave us a report that Jim was slowly returning to normal and his outlook was good. He was walking with minimal assistance and he could talk haltingly, but understandably. His mental processes were continually improving.

Was this just a result of good rehabilitation skills on the healthcare providers' part or was it the result of parents' faith and optimism? I don't have the answer, but it warrants questioning why some patients who have identical problems do well and others do not. Faith and positive attitudes may have a lot more to do with recovery and healing than we realize. We know that the body and the mind are closely interrelated, one affecting the other.

This suggests that nurses' attitudes toward patients and their recovery can also play an important part in this process. Our faith in God and how we show His concern and love for our patients is as essential as the physical care provided.

Check your attitude before interacting with a patient. Be sure you are not distracted with other things or the other stresses of the day. Focus on patients' well being while you are with them and direct your attention solely on them. In this way, their ability to recover and regain wellness will be maximized. Pray in faith that your patients will regain wellness and that their attitudes will also remain positive. God tells us to let Him carry our burdens for us. A positive attitude based on faith in God goes a long way in recovering from illness and injury.

"And the prayer of faith will save ths sick and the Lord will raise him up. And if he has committed sins, he will be forgiven."[1]

David Gerstle

Never, Never, Never, Never, Give Up

...unless God has clearly shown you otherwise.

His quiet, unassuming manner, large "teddy bear" like build and shy smile endeared José not just to me but to all the faculty. To say he was a "favorite" would be quite accurate.

To be a nurse was his goal and he set about his nursing education with great determination. Life is seldom without its difficulties and José was not exempt. Working full time to pay for his tuition and help support his emigrant mother and father took its toll.

Entering my office dressed so neatly and fashionably and with his shy smile hovering around his lips, he simply said "I need your help." Thus began a friendship and journey neither of us could have ever anticipated.

Regular study sessions were scheduled. Even with his tight schedule José was always prompt with his appointments and his aspiration for nursing and appetite for learning never wavered. José seemed to have a good grasp of the concepts of nursing, but testing was his nemesis. It was not without its "ups and downs" that the first semester of nursing (fundamentals of nursing) was finally behind us. I say "us" because in my business of "assisted learning" it feels like an "us" effort since I take it rather personally if a struggling but faithful student does not do well.

The next semester José did not fair so well. His heavy work load and family responsibilities really took its toll. He had to accompany his parents, who spoke very little English, to whatever business had to be accomplished, such as doctor visits, car repairs, purchases, and often had to arbitrate when job difficulties arose for his parents. He felt he had to continue to work full time at a well known baking company to help his family financially.

To make a long story short (as the saying goes) many of the rough spots were smoothed out after he repeated his first med/surg course and cut his work load to half time. Even with the "ups and downs" and discouraging struggles, José graduated with a very decent grade point average. Of course, it was quite a celebration for all of us, his family, friends, classmates and faculty.

The next hurdle was passing the NCLEX (national licensing exam). In the summers I assist students prepare for this examination. As usual José was very faithful with his appointments and practice questions. With great trepidation and anxiety and *prayer* José sat for the exam. The results...not so good.

To cheer him up I said "Lets look on the bright side you can take the exam again in ninety days and we will just practice more and more NCLEX practice questions." This we did. With the ninety days up, he sat for the exam again. The results...bad news again.

"Well, José we are going to keep at this and in ninety days you can take the exam again." I learned that phase well by repeating it every ninety days over the next three years. I also went through the grieving process with José. After each failure José would say, "I feel like the end of the world has come." Then he would shut the door to his room and not talk to anyone for a few days pleading with God to give him wisdom and guidance on what to do. He asked God, "Do You want me to be nurse?" Though he felt the end of the world had come for him, José remarked that something deep down in his soul continued to encourage him that nursing was still the direction God wanted him to go.

After four or so failures, José (who had continued working at his bakery job) decided even if he had to work as an orderly, the hospital work might help him. A guardian angel in the form of a nurse manager named Sue immediately saw José's potential. He was neat, professional, had good critical thinking skills and eager to learn. After a few weeks of orderly work, Sue had José work as a nurse tech and then elevated him to work as a graduate nurse under the supervision of a RN preceptor in anticipation of his passing the NCLEX exam he was to take again in ninety days.

With the ninety days up, some excellent hospital experience behind him and continued practice sessions with me and at home on his computer and much encouragement and many prayers, José went to take the exam in his most optimistic mood. Results...depressing. The good news was Sue, the nurse manager, still had faith in José's potential and continued to let him work under the supervision of a RN. He was respected and well liked by the nursing staff as well as physicians, patients and their families.

Let's fast forward to two more failures (seven altogether) and three years after graduation. The time limit was up with just one more chance in this particular state. By now José was reviewing and practicing questions on his own with just an occasional session from me...mostly just before sitting for the exam. I hadn't heard from José for a while, so I did not know his next scheduled exam date when I went on vacation. Returning home there was a message on my voice mail from José asking to meet with me for a few study sessions before he took the exam again on May 22. The date now was May 31. Immediately calling José, I found him in a very optimistic mood saying he had taken the 265 questions in less then the five-hour limit. Now he was looking up his status on the computer every day but felt it was probably too soon to know the results.

A few days later, on a Monday, when by all accounts his active status should have shown up on the computer if he had passed and it still read "unapproved candidate." Both our moods changed to gloom. However, recalling how many prayers went up in José's behalf over those trying years from friends, family, faculty, and nurses at the hospital did give "us" a glimmer of hope.

The morning after that gloomy Monday, I received a call from José, "We did it" was all he could get out at the moment. When he regained his composure, I asked him what his first thoughts were when he saw his "active" status on the computer screen. Humorously he replied, "Now I don't have to sit in front of that computer and answer practice questions anymore!"

Coming by to show me the printout of his "active status" from the computer, he commented, "I feel I am the most blessed nurse around! I have had so much support from faculty, family, fellow nurses and, of course, God. I can see how all the studying and reviewing have given me an edge many other nurses do not have. For with each failure I had to study and review more and now I have a great base of knowledge that has made me very comfortable with my practice of nursing." He added, "I have no regrets, just thankfulness that the Lord has been with me through those trying years."

Jesus' promise to his disciples "I'll always be with you, even until the end of the world." Matthew 28:20 is very real to José. Is it real to you? It can be if we trust his word.

Bonnie Hunt

The Virtue of Observation

It was one of their first nursing clinicals and still unsure of themselves, Lynn and Jan were delighted to be assigned the same patient, that way they felt they could pool their limited knowledge and resources. The patient, Mr. Howe, was an easily confused gentleman in his late seventies. After introducing themselves, Lynn took his temperature, counted his pulse and respirations, then Jan took his blood pressure. Next, they took turns following their assessment instructions. Using their pen lights, they checked Mr. Howe's pupils, using their stethoscope they checked breath sounds, then abdominal sounds, then felt for pedal pulses. With the assessment completed, the girls chatted with Mr. Howe asking about his health history and about his family while they waited for the breakfast tray to arrive. When the breakfast tray did arrive, Lynn spread Mr. Howe's toast with jam, while Jan opened his juice and silverware package and placed the napkin on his lap. Drinking his orange juice and consuming the scrambled eggs and toast with gusto, the girls noted that Mr. Howe did not suffer from a poor appetite.

After he finished breakfast, the girls had planned to give him his bed bath but decided to provide mouth care first. They looked in the bedside table for toothbrush, toothpaste and emesis basin. There was none. They looked on the over the bed table, none. They searched on top of and in each drawer of a chest of drawers that was in the room to no avail. The bathroom possessed none of the items either. Finally they asked Mr. Howe if he knew where his toothbrush was..."no he didn't."

Jan went to the supply room and retrieved a new set of mouth care supplies. Now they set up a glass of water and emesis basin; then put toothpaste on the toothbrush and handed it to Mr. Howe. Instead of taking the toothbrush with paste as expected, he startled them by saying, "How can I brush my teeth, when you forgot to put them in this morning?"

Even though Lynn and Jan's classmates had a big chuckle over the incident, they lamented, "What kind of nurses are we going to be if we can't even notice a patient doesn't have teeth?"

It took a few days, but the girls began to see the incident as a catalyst for improving their assessment skills and were encourage by looking at Galatians 6:9 in a very practical way, "Let's not become tired of doing good, for in time, we'll reap (better assessment skills) if we don't give up."

Bonnie Hunt

Disillusioned

"You need to write a devotional on disillusionment," sighed Brandi, a recent nursing graduate in orientation at a children's emergency department, who knew I was writing devotional stories for nurses. "No one told me it would be like this. I had no idea I would feel so inadequate. And to think I thought God wanted me to be a nurse!" "What do you want me to write?" I inquired.

"Let me tell you what happened to me in just one shift, the one I worked yesterday. First I went to the PYXIS (a medicine and equipment dispensing machine) and pulled out a SPLINT and brought it to the room where my preceptor was waiting for the SLING she had requested. Keeping everyone waiting I had to run back return the splint and again key into the PYXIS for a SLING and bring it back to my "harried" preceptor. Next, we were trying to start an IV on a very fragile child and missed. I got a new IV needle for my preceptor to try again. She successfully "hit" the vein and asked me to hand her the "T" connector and tubing. "Oh no!" I screamed (to myself). I had put the used needle with 'T' connector in the sharps box and thrown the tubing in the trash. There was my preceptor putting pressure on the vein so it wouldn't bleed out the needle and I was having to run to the PYXIS again to get the new equipment. Unfortunately, there was someone replacing the supplies in the PYXIS and did not feel the same urgency that I felt and made me wait until she was finished.

Next, I was to give directions for a child to go to nuclear medicine; mistakenly, I gave the parents the directions to X-ray. Later I had to transport a child with her mother in tow to nuclear medicine. I was reading the signs to make sure I was going in the right direction and pushed the gurney right into a cart in the hallway jarring the child. I know that mother wondered if I knew what I was doing." Brandi continued, "Do you think Satan is trying to discourage me? On top of all this the nurses are so critical of each other and the other health care providers. My mother warned me that 'nurses eat their young.' I feel all eaten up."

It was no smiling matter to Brandi, but I couldn't help but smile thinking that every nurse alive could probably relate a similar tale of horror.

As faculty, we encourage dedication and competency and teach to a high standard. The result, graduates who enter the real work world with a great deal of idealism and a desire to be competent, compassionate nurses. However, often after I worked a shift reminisce of Brandi's woes, I would suffer a tinge of guilt that we were indeed throwing these innocent young men and women to the sharks. But then I would be buoyed up as I would read "philosophy of nursing" papers, a Nursing Concepts class assignment. It is inspiring to have a fresh and creative look of nursing through the words of these nursing hopefuls. One in particular inspired me and renewed my dedication to be that competent, compassionate nurse we so desire for our students. This young man started his philosophy paper out by saying the Health Care Industry would be worthless without one component: THE NURSE and then went on to write..."Whether it be a mother feeding her child, a son shaving the face of his aged father, an ICU nurse interpreting clinical signs and symptoms of a fresh trauma victim, or a nurse practitioner overworked in an under developed rural, all have one philosophy in common, a commitment to care for others.

Nursing is not a piece of paper, or a few letters after your name, or a white uniform; it is a mind set, a commitment to the care of others. This most basic of abilities bestowed on us is a responsibility that represents symbols of God's love; a devoted pair of hands for His work to be ministered through." Inspired? I was! I shared this philosophy paper with Brandi.

Then Brandi ended our conversation with "All I really want to do is be a really good nurse!" We talked about how hopefully the good days will out weigh the bad days and to always keep in mind that "With God, anything is possible."[1] Also, the Apostle Paul encourages us "Let's not become tired of doing good, for in time, we'll reap the spiritual harvest if we don't give up."[2]

Bonnie Hunt

Body Image Aerobics

Dr. Curtis, an orthopedic surgeon, was sitting at the nurses' station when he received an emergency page on his beeper.

"That's the emergency room. I wonder what they have down there." Dr. Curtis remarked as he punched in the numbers on the telephone. After a few minutes, he hung up the phone.

"I need to get down there, so I'll finish my rounds later," he told me as he got up to leave.

"They have a very bad degloving injury to a young woman who works at one of the nearby factories. They said her right hand is badly mangled." he continued.

Dr. Curtis was a hand specialist and he could do wonders with severe injuries. A degloving injury usually resulted from working on industrial equipment in which the skin and underlying tissue are literally pulled away from the bones just as a glove is removed from the hand. Many times fingers or toes are lost in the trauma. The victim is often left with diminished function of the affected limb.

A while later Dr. Curtis returned to the floor to finish seeing his patients.

"I am going to surgery as soon as I am done. It is going to take a while to do the repairs to the patient's hand. Hopefully I can save some of her fingers and thumb."

We would be getting the patient on the orthopedic unit after she was recovered from anesthesia in the Post Anesthesia Care Unit (PACU). This patient would require a lot of care and monitoring of her circulation status of the affected hand. At the time I did not know the amount of emotional care this patient would require before she left our floor.

Inspiration PRN: Stories About Nurses

The patient's name was Monica. It was about four in the afternoon when she was admitted to our floor. The PACU nurse and a transporter pushed her gurney down the hall to room 335 being careful not to bump into the doorway as they navigated the corners of the room. Monica was still drowsy from the anesthesia and would be for the next several hours. She had a large bandage on her right hand with just two fingertips sticking out of the Kerlex gauze dressing. The nail beds were pale but warm. We propped up her arm on several pillows to prevent any swelling.

After checking her vital signs, circulation, and IVs, we raised the rails on the bed and left the room. Once at the nurses' station, the PACU nurse gave report on the patient. She said the surgery had gone well and there were no problems during the patient's time in PACU. Dr. Curtis could not save three fingers and there was a lot of skin and tissue lost in the injury. A skin graft had been placed over the wound, but further grafting would be needed as the wound healed.

We knew from the extent of the injury that a lot of rehabilitation would be needed to gain function of that hand.

Over the next several days, Dr. Curtis and the nursing staff carefully monitored the progress of healing. The nurses were diligent in assessing circulation and monitoring for any signs of infection. Monica's pain was assessed and controlled with pain medication as often as she needed it. Her physical healing was progressing without complication. However, Monica's injury left an even deeper emotional wound. Depression over the loss of the function of her hand, which led to the loss of income, overtook her. Being a young and beautiful woman, the now mangled but healing hand was quite ugly to her. She became ashamed of her appearance as well as of herself as a person. Even though she could now leave her room and walk around the nursing unit,

Inspiration PRN: Stories About Nurses

she chose to remain in her room. She refused to let friends and family in to visit and would only talk to the nursing staff and the surgeon.

Because of the extent of the injury and the need for intense physical therapy, Monica was allowed to remain in the hospital for monitoring and pain control. As time went on, her trust in the nurses grew and she began to talk about how she felt about her disfiguring injury.

"I feel so ugly and now I am just worthless!" "I was working at the factory job so I could go to college and now that is just a dream." she lamented.

Monica expressed how she just couldn't face people; yet being a very social person she missed being around other people besides the nursing staff. As we talked, a bond began to form between Monica and me. As the charge nurse, I would check on her every day and make "rounds" with Dr. Curtis so she knew me quite well by now. I decided that it might be time to suggest to Monica that we needed to develop a plan for her to get out of her room and be around more people. The first steps would be gradual like walking to the nurses' station and talking to the nurses and then work up to walking to the physical therapy department and getting her therapy there instead of in her room. The next step would be to go to the cafeteria for meals and then to sit in the lobby each day.

Monica was quite skeptical at first, but then agreed to the plan. That afternoon, she appeared at the nurses' station and talked to me. I involved a couple of other nurses in the conversation as the opportunity presented itself. Each day thereafter she left her room more and more. She ate several times in the cafeteria and went to the lobby once a day. Progress was being made.

One day a flyer was posted announcing an aerobics class being offered to the community and hospital staff. It was to be held at the hospital in one of the conference rooms. This seemed like a good opportunity for Monica to stretch her wings a little more and attend the class. Although she could not use her hand, she could participate in the less strenuous exercises and most importantly be around people. It was also a good environment because many people are self-conscious in an aerobics class anyway, so Monica certainly would not be alone in her feelings. Before suggesting this to Monica, I cleared the idea with Dr. Curtis. He gave his approval but with caution about protecting her hand. It was healed enough now that there would be little danger of injury.

When I suggested the aerobics class to Monica, she was hesitant. Thinking on my feet, I told her that several of the nurses including myself would go with her. She liked that idea and agreed to do so only if the staff attended with her. I hadn't asked anybody yet, but I had faith in my peers and I knew I would get volunteers. After talking to Monica, I returned to the nurses' station and began recruiting. I didn't have to bribe too much and most of the nurses said they would go if I went. Amazingly, quite a number signed up for the classes.

The aerobic classes were held in the early evening so I returned to the hospital and signed Monica out for the class. She was quite self-conscious but was dressed in sweats and ready to go.

"Everyone is going to stare at me. I am going to stand out." she said.

"Well, probably no more than at everyone else. Have you looked at the nursing staff lately?" I joked.

Monica laughed nervously, "I'm glad you guys are coming with me."

As we entered the room where the class was being held, the other nursing staff members greeted Monica. The instructor then told us to form lines so we could begin exercising. The music began to play as the instructor worked through the various aerobic steps. Fortunately the class was for beginners and not too strenuous. The class was intent on following the instructor and did not seem to even notice Monica's hand.

By the end of class, Monica was tired but had a smile on her face. I asked her how she felt about the class now.

"It wasn't bad at all. In fact it felt good. No one was staring at me like I thought. They were probably staring at you; you are not the most coordinated soul I have ever seen." she teased.

"Hey, I resemble that remark!" I responded as we both laughed.

Each week that we attended the aerobics class, Monica became more confident and less self-conscious. She spent her last days in the hospital visiting other patients and giving them encouragement. She shared with them how she was coping with her injury and her recovery. She had made quick progress in her rehabilitation through physical therapy and could now continue on an outpatient basis. It was a tearful goodbye when Monica was dismissed from the hospital. She thanked us for our care and support. She was even more grateful we went with her to the aerobics class! She was now well on her way to physical and emotional health.

How often do we as nurses lose confidence and become self-conscious? It may be related to professional responsibilities or family responsibilities or the overwhelming combined responsibility of both. We may tend to shut people out and isolate ourselves. Sometimes when support is offered, we do not accept it and try to cope on our own. However, God never intended for us to bear our burdens alone. He never intended for us to see ourselves as worthless or ugly; each of us is a child of the King. God has invited us to come to Him in need and ask for help in our prayers. We must wait on Him to answer them.

"Wait on the Lord, be of good courage, and he shall strengthen thy heart: wait I say, on the Lord."[1]

"Fear thou not: for I am with thee: be not dismayed; for I am thy God: I will strengthen thee; yea, I will help thee; yea, I will uphold thee with the right hand of my righteousness."[2]

Post-script: Several weeks later, Monica came to visit the nurses to show them her new prosthesis for her hand. It was quite natural looking and helped Monica to feel even more normal. Dr. Curtis paid for the prosthesis himself since she could not afford it and the insurance company would not pay for such a prosthesis. He even hired her to work in his office. Monica also decided to become a nurse and was pursuing scholarships for entrance into a school of nursing at the time this story occurred.

David Gerstle

Ain't Gonna Do It!

"I'm not getting up! Ain't gonna do it!"

Richard, a patient two days post-op lumbar laminectomy and fusion, had been fitted with his back corset. It was time for him to get out of his hospital bed for the first time since surgery. Richard was a healthy young man in his twenties who had injured his back in an industrial accident. Prior to surgery, he was anxious, but no more than was usual for patients undergoing this procedure. Now Richard was wound up as tight as a rubber band stretched across the Golden Gate bridge. That's anxious!

I was standing by his bed with another nurse to help Richard stand and then take a few steps. He was lying on his back looking up at us. His jaw was set and his forehead was furrowed. He was glaring at me.

"Richard, we really need to get you up. It is important for you to starting walking several times a day. You'll even feel better."

"I told you I am not getting up! You can just forget it."

I tried to reason with him. I tried to bring humor into it. I used all of the motivating ideas I knew, but nothing I said changed his mind. For some reason he did not want to get up.

"Richard, if we come back later, will you get up?"

"No, I ain't gonna do it!"

"Are you hurting? We gave you some medicine so you would be more comfortable when you stood up."

"I'm not hurting and I'm NOT getting up!"

Now, I am not advocating the actions I took next, but I intuitively knew that Richard needed to stand up now. I felt quite convinced and without hesitation I told the patient we were going to assist him to a standing position.

"No, you're not! I am going to report you to the hospital president" he said trembling with anger. Or, was it fear?

"What is your last name, Dave? I am reporting you!"

"It's Gerstle" I said as I pointed to my badge.

I continued in my quest to get Richard up despite his protests. Obviously, this course of action goes against all principles in nursing and human interaction. While Richard was threatening lawsuits, having my RN license revoked, and cursing, my partner and I helped him to a sitting position.

"Are you hurting? Are you dizzy?"

"No, but you are going to pay for this!" Richard said as we had him sit and take some slow deep breaths.

"Ok, Richard, we are going to stand you up now. We won't let you fall. Just straighten your legs as we lift you and then stand."

"No, don't!" Richard repeated as he stood.

He was almost in tears and his voice was trembling; this time it was certainly due to fear. When he reached the full standing position, his protests and his trembling stopped. He physically relaxed as we stood there together by his bed. A smile even erupted on his face.

"I'm not paralyzed!"

Richard had an incredulous look on his face to add to his smile. We took a few steps forward and then returned him to the bed to sit.

Richard grabbed my right hand with both of his hands and shook it as vigorously as a post-op back surgery patient could.

"Thank you! Thank you! Thank you! I thought I wouldn't be able to walk and I didn't want to find out for sure. Thank you for making me do it."

Fortunately, my intuitiveness led to an accurate assessment of the patient and his needs. I just knew he thought he couldn't walk and the only way to convince him otherwise was to force him to do it. A risky intervention, but sometimes gut decisions are your best guide.

Over the next couple of days, Richard progressed from standing with assistance to walking around the unit several times on his own. He would always greet me with a big smile and thank me again for making him stand up. He was dismissed a day early because he was doing so well. He never did report me to the hospital president.

Richard wasn't really paralyzed, but he thought he was. He was quite capable of walking, but was very afraid that he could not.

Have you ever been mentally or emotionally paralyzed that you believed you could not achieve something? Life can be a scary thing and can also be busy and complicated. We can become overwhelmed with all of its demands and setbacks. This leads to a type of paralysis that prevents us from attempting things that may involve the risk of failure. Many times this causes us to give into the fear and avoid facing challenges that present themselves.

Jesus said that we should not fear things but to depend on Him for He would provide for our needs. He wants us to be confident that if we follow Him, we can succeed. Fear is a natural emotion, yet we should not be so fearful of failure that we are paralyzed. Will we succeed at everything we attempt? No. Will we accomplish anything when we fail? Yes. We will learn what doesn't work and try another avenue.

Thomas Edison failed many times at inventing the light bulb. He learned how not to make a light bulb, which led to his success at finally inventing one that worked. We also will learn that sharing our experiences

Inspiration PRN: Stories About Nurses

of failure with others before we reach success will encourage others who are experiencing failure.

We learn and grow from our experiences thus each of us has something to offer. Each of us can use our talents and experience to help others. Don't allow yourself to avoid challenges and accomplishments because of the fear of failure. Failure is a part of the success process. God invites us to depend on Him. If we fail, take it to Him in prayer. When we succeed, give glory to Him. Don't be paralyzed by fear. Lean on the Lord and take that first step.

"Strengthen the weak hands and make firm the feeble knees. Say to those who are fearful-hearted, be strong, do not fear! Behold, your God will come with vengeance with the recompense of God; He will come and save you."[1]

David Gerstle

Florence

She was born with a "silver spoon in her mouth," so the saying goes. Her wealthy parents, the Nightingale's, had homes in London and in the English countryside. Ambitions for their daughters were the "good life"...social events, travel, needlework, music, and drawing.

Parthenope, one of their daughters, took to the good life like a duck to water, but this was not so for Florence; she was a very unhappy camper. She wanted to be a nurse. This unconventional ambition horrified her parents. Why only the poor took their sick to the hospital and "privileged" young ladies would never work in institutions that were so loathsome and unsanitary.

Undaunted by the conventional wisdom of the day, Florence tried to persuade her parents to let her work in a nearby hospital. With her parents' adamant refusal of the idea, Florence settled into a miserable, depressed state, longing for a life of service to relieve the "sufferings of man," and care for those with disease. It was during this time that Florence rejected a marriage proposal stating she had a "passionate nature which requires satisfaction." This nature could not be satisfied "by spending a life with him (her suitor) in making society and arranging domestic things." Her refusal to marry further infuriated her parents. To boost her sagging spirits, Florence covertly read books about nursing and hospitals. She came upon information about a reputable hospital in Kaiserswerth, Germany that was run by deaconesses that were skilled in nursing. Elated, she secretly cherished thoughts that one day she would be able to train as a nurse there.

It was a "stroke of luck" or more then likely "providence" that Florence was invited by family friends

Inspiration PRN: Stories About Nurses

to vacation with them in Europe. They were aware of her secret interest in the Kaiserswerth hospital and indicated they would arrange a visit to Kaiserswerth if she accompanied them on this trip to Europe. After her visit to Kaiserswerth and observing the routines and techniques by the doctors and nurses for several weeks, Florence returned home "feeling so brave as if nothing could ever vex me again." However, vexation did return. Her parents were furious when they found out she had visited Kaiserswerth. Now they insisted she be a companion to her sister...go for rides in the country, draw, sing, and do needlework. "I have no desire now but to die" wrote Florence in her journal.

About a year after her visit to Kaiserswerth and after many a stormy argument, Florence was 'grudgingly' allowed to return to Kaiserswerth and train as a nurse. The rest is history. After studying at Kaiserswerth, Florence returned to London with the highest of recommendations...for it was said that no one had so thoroughly mastered the art of nursing and passed the exam with so great of distinction as Miss Nightingale. She became superintendent of a London hospital that catered to the "genteel."

Then it was off to the Crimean war where she is credited with saving the lives of thousands of sick and wounded soldiers by improving the sanitary conditions in military field hospitals. Not only was Florence's brilliant administrative abilities demonstrated during her service in the Crimean war, but so was her compassionate nature. Late into the night after her administrative and nursing duties of the day were completed, Florence would light her lamp and make her way to the bedside of wounded soldiers providing comfort and words of encouragement. Thus, she became known as the "lady with the lamp."

After returning to London as a national heroine, Florence spent her time promoting hospital administration and reform and founded the Nightingale School and Home for Nurses. I write this short tribute of Miss Florence Nightingale least we forget to credit her for elevating the quality of nursing education and status of nurses in England as well as here in America that still resonates today.

I once read that Florence felt she was "Called of God" to a life of service. Undaunted by what could have been insurmountable obstacles, her unconventional ambition and her parents' adamant objections, Florence pursued that call. With the bad press nursing is getting, overworked, underpaid, not appreciated, I wonder how many today will have the same tenacity to persevere in the choice to be a nurse under these similar circumstances as Florence encountered?

"And we know that God causes everything to work together for the good of those who love him and are called by Him."[1]

Bonnie Hunt

A Train with No Caboose

The 4-year-old boy's eyes lit up when he saw the wooden train for the first time. "Is it really mine? Can I really keep it?" he exclaimed. His eyes never left the train; as if it might disappear if he should lose sight of it.

"Yes, it really is yours," I replied.

"Oh, boy, oh, boy, thank you, thank you!" the little hospital patient repeated again and again as he played with his toy train. Around and around the bed the train went, with wooden wheels rolling over imaginary tracks.

This toy train isn't just any toy train. First of all, it is a wooden toy train crafted by hand. It has an engine, a coal car, a flat car complete with a load of wooden logs, a boxcar, and a caboose. Another thing that makes this train very special is that it was made and given by someone who simply wanted to give trains away to children who are patients in hospitals.

Several years ago a man whom I'll call Charles was going to an outpatient clinic weekly for chemotherapy to treat cancer. As he waited each week at the clinic, he befriended a little boy who was going there for chemotherapy as well. The two became fast friends. One week Charles brought the boy a wooden train engine. The little boy was just thrilled with the toy. So each week when Charles met the little boy, he would give him another train car.

Charles was looking forward to completing the wooden train for the little boy, and finally the week came for the caboose. He sat down in his usual place at the clinic and waited and waited, but the boy did not come. He went to the reception desk to ask if his young friend had canceled or changed his appointment for the day. One of the nurses explained that the boy had been admitted to the hospital and had died only the day before.

This was a crushing blow to Charles. In addition to feeling the loss of the child, he felt terrible that he didn't get a chance to give the little boy a caboose to finish his train. And now, years later, he gives toy trains to children who are patients, although he insists on giving them *complete* toy trains.

The 4-year-old at the beginning of the story was one of many patients who received a toy train at the hospital where I worked as nurse manager of a pediatric floor. It all began when the train maker came to the Respiratory Therapy Department for pulmonary treatments. He asked if he could bring the trains to be given to the children who are patients.

Upon their admission to the hospital, each child was given a wooden toy train, and a Polaroid picture was taken for the train maker. Many smiles were recorded each week as the trains were handed out, giving comfort to the receiver and giver as well.

Just as this toy train maker wants each child to have a complete train, Jesus wants each of us to have a complete life in Him. Many of us are not complete - we may be physically, emotionally, or spiritually incomplete.

Jesus, the divine maker, has promised that He will return again and make us whole. We must talk to Him daily and allow Him to lead in our lives so that we will be ready to meet Him at His coming. And what a coming that will be! As His followers rise up to meet Him, immortality will replace mortality, physical perfection will replace physical deformities, and eternal joy and happiness will replace emotional turmoil and pain.

Perhaps as all of this is taking place, the toy train maker and the little boy who had suffered from cancer will meet. The man will reach down into his celestial robe and pull out a wooden toy caboose. Giving it to the boy, he might say, "Son, I've been saving this for you when we would meet again in eternity."

Are you ready to let Jesus make you complete?

David Gerstle

Inspiration PRN: Stories About Nurses

PERCEPTIONS

Knifepoint

Being run off the road by a car while riding a motorcycle was not a biker's idea of a fun afternoon. Jerry was on the interstate on his big Harley and enjoying the warm Texas wind as he blew down the road. Fortunately he was in the right lane when the car next to him entered his lane almost hitting him. Jerry saw the car just in time to steer his bike onto the side of the road and out of the way of the car or other traffic. Unfortunately, he was traveling 65 miles per hour and lost control. Hitting the surface hard on his right side, Jerry and the bike went skidding down the shoulder of the road.

The driver of the car stopped and stayed with Jerry after calling 911 for an ambulance and the police. Being in a lot of pain and looking at the wreck of a Harley he now owned, Jerry was not in any mood to hear excuses from the driver.

"I didn't even see you!" the older male driver exclaimed.

"You ran me off the road, man. Are you blind? You better watch your back, I know a few bikers who will be happy to come visit you." Jerry snarled threateningly as he looked over the driver and his car.

"Look, I'm sorry you wrecked." The now frightened driver replied.

He walked back to his car and waited for the police. Jerry was now really hurting from his right leg and the road rash on various places on his right side. The ambulance couldn't arrive soon enough.

After being seen by the emergency physician and the orthopedic surgeon who were on call, Jerry was informed he was going to surgery to have his right tibia-fibula repaired. This news evoked a few choice words

Inspiration PRN: Stories About Nurses

from Jerry and put him in an angrier mood than he was in before. He wasn't in any better mood when we received him postoperatively on the orthopedic unit.

"Have you seen that guy in room 305? He's scary looking. Dave. I think you should take him this shift." Vicki, one of the other nurses on duty with me that evening said.

"He can't be that scary."

"Well, he's a biker and he is not happy to be here. He's cussin' a blue streak."

As a nurse, I had taken care of a number of bikers who had a rough and tumble lifestyle. Most of them had good hearts with rough looking exteriors. Agreeing to take over Jerry's care, I walked into his room and introduced myself. Jerry basically was still groggy from the anesthesia, but definitely still mad about being run off the road. I planned to keep his pain under control for both our sakes. Throughout the evening, we got along well. I showed respect for him by never making him feel like he couldn't handle the pain like a man. We agreed it was a really bad break to his leg and a lesser man wouldn't be able to take it even with pain medication. He seemed in a little better mood by the end of the shift and was now sleeping off and on.

Jerry had to stay in the hospital a few days for antibiotics and physical therapy. After a day off, I was working the day shift. The night shift charge nurse, Robert, met me at the desk and said that the "biker" patient gave him a hard time all night and barely let him in the room.

"He really doesn't like me; and now I just saw a bunch of his friends go into his room. They probably are out to get me."

"Robert, you sound a bit paranoid. After report, you need to go home and get some sleep."

"Paranoid?" he exclaimed. "Did you know he keeps a knife under his pillow?"

This surprised me.

"I will go talk to him and tell him he can't keep a knife in the hospital."

I walked to Jerry's room and before I could enter the doorway, his "biker" friends, all taller and bigger than me and covered with a few tattoos, surrounded me in the hallway. It wasn't exactly a welcome back party as their faces were set in hard menacing lines.

"Not him, not him!" I heard Jerry yelling from his bed. His friends looked over at him as if disappointed they couldn't hit me or threaten me or do something violent.

"He's cool!" Jerry continued, "It's that spooky guy who was here during the night."

Gathering my courage, I pushed past the "Hell's Angels" and went in to talk to Jerry.

"Jerry, what's up with the night nurse? He said you have a knife and you have been hassling him."

Reaching behind his pillow, Jerry pulls out a long hunting knife with a carved wood handle.

"I always sleep with a knife. The places I stay you need to sleep with one eye open and a way to protect yourself. That spooky night guy kept coming in my room without warning. I told him he gave me the "creeps" and I would get him the next time he showed up in my room unannounced."

"What's with the bikers in the hallway?" I asked pointing to his pals.

"Those are my biker brothers. They were going to let "Spooky" know to stay out of my room or get the 'hurt' put on him."

Seeing that I was still standing and knowing that Jerry thought I was cool, I pushed my luck a bit further.

"Jerry, you know you can't keep a knife in the hospital. After your buddies leave (I knew he didn't want to look like a wimp in front of his friends), will you give me you knife? I'll lock it up until you get dismissed."

"No way, man. I've slept with a knife for years."

"Robert only works week-ends and you will be gone before he returns. I'll tell the other nurses to knock before coming in you room at night. Will you give up the knife then?"

"Dude, you've been all right (But am I still cool?). I'll give you the knife later, but you tell everyone who comes in here to knock or make some kind of noise before coming near me. I won't guarantee I won't hit them."

That certainly was better than a knifing. All ended well. No one was stabbed. Robert and I didn't get the "hurt" put on us. The knife was returned to Jerry when he went home and hopefully he never found the driver that put him in the hospital in the first place.

Nurses many times have to deal with patients who have many different emotions including anger and fear. Patients are from all walks of life and many times we may not understand why patients perceive things as they do. As nurses, we must try to understand and not be judgmental. We must follow Christ's example of accepting people where they are.

David Gerstle

Jumping to Conclusions

It had started out as a quiet morning at the nursing home. As I entered the front lobby, the usual residents were at their self-appointed places. Each were in their respective chairs after breakfast in the dining hall and gave me their "Good Mornings" and waves. Mrs. Bryer and Mr. Jones were sitting side by side in their wheelchairs where the nurse assistant had left them until medication time. Mrs. Bryer always grabbed my hand as I greeted them and wouldn't let go until I spent a few minutes with them. A stroke had taken away her ability to speak coherently but it didn't interfere with her "talking" to you anyway. Mr. Jones could speak well and always had something to say. He kept Mrs. Bryer company.

"It's going to be a good day." Mr. Jones said positively as he did every time I saw him.

Yes, it would be a good day. It was going to be a routine predictable good day or so I thought.

After visiting with the pair, I proceeded to the nurses' station and met with the director of nurses. In addition to my hospital position, I "moonlighted" as a RN consultant for two nursing homes. I provided continuing education for the staff as well as advised on the care of the residents. Today, I soon learned the DON was short a medication nurse and had to pass medications.

"I am really going to be busy today!" she informed me.

"Is there anything I can do to help out?" I asked.

"There is one thing that must be done today. Mr. Wright is scheduled for transfer to the VA hospital. I have contacted them and made all of the arrangements. I just need you to call the transport service to take him there."

Inspiration PRN: Stories About Nurses

This was easy enough or should have been. It was just a matter of calling the service and giving a quick report on the patient. The ambulance company that contracted with the city had an emergency service and a non-emergency service. This provided quick response for emergencies as non-emergencies didn't take the emergency ambulances away from true emergencies. The fire department also came to emergency calls team since their stations were throughout the city.

Mr. Wright was a chronic obstructive pulmonary disease (COPD) patient of long standing who needed long-term custodial care. As a veteran, he was entitled to VA care so he had requested moving to that facility.

I went to Mr. Wright's room and let him know I was calling the ambulance for his trip to the VA. I assessed him and noted that he had a rapid pulse. He had been diagnosed with sinus tachycardia several years ago. Medication did not work well slowing his heart and the theophylline he took for his COPD did not help matters. Because of his age, respiratory condition, and seemingly lack of other symptoms caused by the rapid pule, his physician did not try to do anything further to control it. Satisfied he was stable for the move, I called the non-emergency transfer service.

"Dispatcher" intoned the deep voice on the other end.

"Yes, this is Gerstle, RN at Edgewood Nursing Home. We need an ambulance to transfer a resident to the VA hospital."

I gave all of the necessary information for the transfer to the emotionless dispatcher including the patient's medical diagnoses of COPD and sinus tachycardia.

"What are his vitals?" the dispatcher asked disinterestedly.

"Temp is 98.8, pulse 128, respirations 28, BP is..."

"His pulse is what?!" The dispatcher now was alert, his voice excited and rising in pitch."

"It's 128, but it has been rapid for years. He is stable and his BP is 122 over..." Interrupted again.

"This man is going to code. I'm calling 911 and have an emergency response team come."

"No, don't do that! He is stable. I checked him myself. His vitals are abnormal but he is fine."

Too late. I heard the dispatcher over the phone calling in the "emergency."

"I have a possible cardiac at Edgewood Nursing Home. His vitals are..." was heard clearly as Junior MD alerted the paramedic cavalry.

I continued to protest. I tried to explain again that the man was stable. No chest pain, no difficulty breathing. I even tried to pull rank on "Panic Paul" and tell him I was a RN. Nothing worked, he was convinced the man was at death's door. I think he was either in the wrong job or he was terribly bored with his "non-emergency dispatcher" job.

Knowing how quickly the fire department and ambulance could respond, I rushed to Mr. Wright's room to let him know he was about to have a whole lot of visitors.

"Mr. Wright, you might be seeing some firemen and paramedics in a few minutes, but don't panic. It's a bit of a false alarm."

"Ok, was something on fire?"

"Only the dispatcher."

"What?"

"Just kidding" I said. "The dispatcher just misunderstood that you just needed a ride to the VA."

Next I went to the nurses' station and warned the staff of what had happened and what was about to occur. A moment later the sound of sirens was heard at the front entrance. I headed to the lobby and was greeted by

Inspiration PRN: Stories About Nurses

a squad of firemen dressed in full gear and armed with oxygen and first aid kits.

"Where's the fire?" Mr. Jones asked as they rushed inside.

Mrs. Bryer tried to grab one of the fireman's hand.

"Wait, wait!" I pleaded. "There's been a mistake."

"Where's the victim?" asked a fireman as his squad gathered beside him.

I wanted to say he was standing in front of him; instead I began to explain the situation only to be interrupted now by the paramedics rushing through the door. They wanted to save somebody. You could see it in their eyes.

The paramedics wanted the location of the victim as well. Surrounded by firemen and paramedics, I explained the situation of the dispatcher jumping to conclusions. You could almost see the disappointment in their eyes.

"Well, we're here now so we need to check him out." said one of the paramedics.

We all walked down the hall to Mr. Wright's room. The firemen wanted to see for themselves that there was no victim. The paramedics attached the Lifepac cardiac monitor and were soon convinced Mr. Wright was stable for transport.

"So, are you going to take him to the VA?" I asked.

"No, we are the emergency ambulance service. There is no emergency here" said the paramedic.

He suppressed the laugh that was coming out in response to the irony of the situation.

However he did call the "non-emergency dispatcher" for me and explained that it was best to replace jumping to conclusions with level headedness and better telephone triage. Mr. Wright finally went to the VA without the benefits of lights and sirens.

Have you ever jumped to conclusions and then regretted it later? How about making assumptions that were unfounded? I know I have done both. Sometimes it only means some embarrassment. Other times these conclusions and assumptions are negative and destructive. They lead to unnecessary worry and energy to resolve situations that don't even exist. Damaged relationships and hurt feelings may also occur especially when one assumes how another feels or thinks instead of actually listening to one another's true feelings. People want to be understood and valued. This doesn't occur when we make our own surmising. Perhaps this why the Bible states "Do not judge less you be judged." We are not good judges. We don't see every thing (perhaps because we jump to conclusions), thus imperfect judgment leads to bad decisions. We assume imminent heart failure when there is only a rapid beat.

"Judge not, that you be not judged. For with what judgment you judge, you will be judged, and with the same measure you use, it will be measured back to you."[1]

David Gerstle

You Know I (Can) Dance

The seemingly frail patient barely occupied the hospital bed she was in. Her slight form was just discernable under the covers. Mrs. Appleby had fallen and fractured her hip at home. She had her hip pinned the day before since it was not a severe break. Approaching the bed slowly so not to frighten her, I quietly said, "Good Morning." Peeking out from under the covers, an elderly brown face turned to me. Blinking her eyes a couple of times, Mrs. Appleby smiles brightly and says "Why, good morning to you!" in a genteel Southern accent.

I immediately had the impression she was not as frail as I had thought after all. I helped her wash her face and brush her teeth as the breakfast trays were being passed out. She was quite alert since the surgeon had used a spinal anesthesia to perform the surgery. Mrs. Appleby chattered as she ate and I did parts of my assessment. After breakfast, I returned to finish up the paperwork that wasn't yet completed upon her admission. I then assisted her to a chair to sit for a few minutes. She was doing very well and tolerated it easily.

Mrs. Appleby loved to talk. The surgeon came in and I gave him a quick report. He and his assistant stayed a little bit as Mrs. Appleby explained to us she was 95 years old and had never been in a hospital before, not even when she was born. Her grandparents had been slaves and her parents lived on the same plantation as freemen at the turn of the century. Mrs. Appleby was born in their home there. She grew up picking cotton and tending gardens as a child and a teenager until she married and moved away.

Being African-American and living in the South during those years was a hardship on her. Yet, she explained that she always had an optimistic attitude toward life. She learned to appreciate the good things. This she attributed to her good health and long years.

Her audience was captivated by her story and her sweet Southern voice. "What else do you think has given you good health?" we asked.

"Well" Mrs. Appleby drawled, as she put her finger to her chin, pondering the question. "I don't smoke. I don't drink either. I don't eat much meat. Sometimes I eat chicken, but we could hardly afford meat when I was growing up. I eat a lot of beans and greens and 'taters. I do love cornbread though. I eat fruit like apples and peaches, whatever is in season. Once in a while, I eat a sweet. Sometimes, I just like cornbread and buttermilk with sugar on top."

We all made a face at the mention of cornbread and buttermilk.

"It's gooooood!" Mrs. Appleby exclaimed, "Try it some time."

"What else do you do?" I asked.

"I walk every day. I used to walk three or four miles a day, but now I just walk around my neighborhood."

"You live by yourself?" I asked.

"Sure, I can take care of myself. But my granddaughter visits me every day too. Good thing, I guess, since she was the one who found me when I fell." Mrs. Appleby laughed at the thought.

"One more thing I want to ask you. What is the most important thing you want to be able to do when you get out of the hospital?"

She broke out in a big grin, "I have to get back to my dancing."

Dancing? A 95-year-old woman dancing?

"You dance?"

"Sure, honey, every week at the senior center. I can 'cut a rug' too. Wait 'til I get better; I'll show you."

And she did. The day before she was discharged, she walked out of her room with her walker and the physical therapist. Stopping me in the hall, she showed me some slow but most excellent dance steps.

Perhaps, we all can learn some things from Mrs. Appleby about good health and longevity:

>Be optimistic   Eat lots of vegetables and fruit
>Don't drink   Eat few sweets
>Don't smoke   Walk every day
>and DANCE.

David Gerstle

Instructions

I was making rounds checking on my nursing students and their preceptors when I heard "Mrs. Hunt! Mrs. Hunt! You won't believe what just happened!" "Oh no," I moaned inwardly.

"What happened?" "One of my patients, Mrs. Thomson, is going for surgery tomorrow morning and an order was left for her to scrub her abdomen three times with the antiseptic soap, Hibiclens. My preceptor handed me a Styrofoam cup to fill with Hibiclens from the floor stock. I filled the cup and took it to the Mrs. Thomson's room. She was preoccupied with unpacking and visiting with her family, so I briefly explained that after her family left she was to shower and scrub her abdomen three times with the solution that I would leave on the rim of the tub. After her family left, she went into the bathroom and saw the cup sitting there. She said she paused for a moment and tried to remember what I had told her...then looking at the solution in the cup she picked it up and drank it."

"Then what did you do?" I inquired. Sue continued, "I hurried and told my preceptor. The preceptor called the pharmacist and he indicated probably no harm was done. Then she said he laughed and told us to watch her closely for bubbles."

Sue moaned, "Now I have to fill out an incident report." After filling out the incident report Sue sighed, "Well! I learned at least two things to day...make sure the patient understands my instructions and don't put any thing in a cup that isn't for drinking."

This incident brought back a memory of many years ago. This sweet elderly couple stood looking at me nodding and smiling as I explained about the wife's medication. The wife had come to the clinic complaining of episodes of shortness of breath and difficulty breathing. The resident had ordered aminophylline suppositories *PRN* (as needed).

"She gets frightened when she can't breathe and it scares me too," explained the husband in a heavy Hebrew accent. "She needs medicine."

"This is what these suppositories are for," I instructed. With hand gestures and speaking slowly I continued my instructions, "When she has difficulty breathing you take off the wrapper and have her insert it in her rectum." I cautioned she was only to use the suppositories when she had an episode of shortness of breath or difficulty breathing. Both smiled and nodded then smiled again and nodded and seemed pleased with the medication I handed them from our clinic supply.

Two weeks later I spotted the elderly couple as they were being ushered to a room for their appointment. Greeting them I inquired if the medication had helped. With a half nod and a semi smile the husband replied, "Helped some. They were too big for her to swallow so she had to break them in half and chew them." Oooh no! I thought and then proceeded to ask a silly question, "Didn't she complained they tasted bad?" "Sometimes she did," the husband replied. I don't remember who but someone came to my rescue with a word that they would understand on how to administer the medication.

The Psalmist reveals that "(God) will teach (instruct) you the way that you should go: and (He) will keep (His) eye on you and guide you along safe paths."[1]

When I pay attention to God's instructions, my path is safe. But often I find myself like my patients...too preoccupied, don't pause long enough, too comfortable with the familiar, and sometimes I even nod and smile and pretend I understand. The results...I drink a solution intended for scrubbing and I chew distasteful medicine that should have been administered by another method.

Bonnie Hunt

Don't Run

"Hi! I am Jennifer Saxton, a student nurse, and I will be taking care of you today. I am going to do a head-to-toe assessment. First, I am going to place a stethoscope on your chest and listen to your lungs and heart." Jennifer listened carefully and commented all sounds seemed to be normal. Then she explained about listening to his bowel sounds. For the neuro check she instructed her patient to grip both of her hands, to touch his nose, to smile, etc. Her patient, Mr. Webber, being blind, made Jennifer alert to the fact she should explain her every move. He was a diabetic and had a large infected ulceration on his right leg. Jennifer told him she was going to examine his leg ulcer, which she did without comment but noted to herself it "looked good" and seemed to be healing well. Then Jennifer told Mr. Webber she was going to get his breakfast tray.

When Jennifer reentered Mr. Webber's room, she did not introduce herself again assuming he would recognize her voice. Placing the breakfast tray on his "over the bed" table, Jennifer took the plastic wrap off the silverware and the lid off his hot drink. Not recognizing Jennifer's voice as she had assumed, Mr. Webber asked, "Who is your supervisor? There was a student in here looking at my wound and it bothered her so I don't want her taking care of me."

Jennifer said, "My first instinct was to run out of the room as fast as I could and find my nursing instructor and cry 'My patient doesn't want me to take care of him.'"

Instead with all the composure she could muster up Jennifer replied, "I am the student that looked at your wound and it didn't bother me; it looked good and seemed to be healing nicely. But if you would like I will get another student to come in and take care of you." "Oh! If it didn't bother you then it's o.k." informed Mr. Webber. Even though still feeling a little embarrassed over the situation, Jennifer continued with her care for Mr. Webber. It did not take long for Jennifer and Mr. Webber to get into some good conversations from the mundane to the spiritual. They found they had many common interests. Jennifer stayed with Mr. Webber most of the lab but always introduced her self every time she entered his room. At the end of the shift Mr. Webber commented he enjoyed her and appreciated the good care she had provided and hoped she would be his nurse the next day. "It felt good to know I did not run away from what seemed like a bad situation for me. It actually turned out to be a good experience, one I will always remember," mused Jennifer.

How many times have we, like Jennifer, wanted to run from an unpleasant situation? Particularly if a criticism is directed at us personally. It does take a lot of composure to work though a tough situation. From where does that inter strength come?

Hopefully, we will be like the Psalmist David who when in a tough situation (which seemed to be most of the time) would always cry out pleading to the Lord for help. Help did come for David proclaimed "I waited patiently for the lord to help me, and He listened and heard my cry."[1]

So it is with confidence that David tells us, "The Lord guides those who depend on Him and gives them the help they need...The Lord helps the righteous and gives them support in times of trouble."[2]

When we draw our inner strength from the right source as we face tough situations, perhaps we, too, can say as Jennifer did, "It actually turned out to be a good experience, one I will always remember."

Bonnie Hunt

COMFORT MEASURES

Painful Lessons

Before me on my desk is a clever little ruler. It has number markings from zero to five which is not so clever...but the smiley faces scattered along these markings is an inventive way of allowing a child to describe the intensity of pain being experienced. Number zero face has a very bright smile, no pain, then the smile changes to a more somber expression until the number five face has a furrowed brow with tears streaming from the eyes, "bad" pain. Usually when nurses assess the intensity of pain experienced by an adult, we may simply ask "On a scale zero to ten, zero being no pain and ten being the worst pain you can imagine, how would you rate your pain?"

Also in my possession is another pain assessment ruler that has numbered blocks of color...number zero a white block, indicates no pain, number one a blue colored block, represents mild, annoying, nagging pain and on up the scale of blocks until number five, a red block represents excruciating, torturing, crushing, tearing pain. This is a great tool for assessing pain for those who know their colors but not numeric values. I remember the days before these clever, resourceful devices were available and view these rulers a more accurate way of assessing the pain of my patients then the nurse's subjective evaluation of muscle tension or tears. But beware! These clever little devices do not tell the whole story.

Elderly Mrs. Jones pushed her call bell and requested "something for pain." It had been four hours since her last dose of Demerol. Nurse Nancy Brown checked the chart and noted that Mrs. Jones had been receiving Demerol about every four hours since her surgery (removal of a small benign abdominal mass) two days ago, even though she had an order for a less potent oral analgesic. Thinking it unusual that Mrs. Jones was still requiring such a strong pain medication, Nancy asked Mrs. Jones about her pain. Mrs. Jones simply replied, "It's pretty bad." "Where is your pain?" Nancy inquired. Mrs. Jones pointed in the direction of her buttocks. Turning Mrs. Jones over Nancy found embedded in the middle of her left buttock a plastic cap (like one used to cover a plastic cup). Viola! With the removal of the cap the pain disappeared. Now it was only occasionally that she requested "something" for mild abdominal discomfort. Sadly, it seemed no one had bothered inquiring as to the location of Mrs. Jones' pain. Yes, Mrs. Jones had been up ambulating, yes Mrs. Jones' bed linens had been changed, and yes Mrs. Jones had given herself a bath. But the cap was so imbedded that it had just stayed in place during all those tasks.

It was Mrs. Westen's third cholecystectomy postoperative day. Instead of her pain diminishing she was indicating her pain was a ten and was requiring stronger and stronger doses of a pain medicine. Mrs. Westen became confused, she did not recognize her son, did not know where she was, and adamantly refused to ambulate. The staff attributed this to her being old and to the effects of narcotics.

Shauna, a niece, came by for a visit and was alarmed to see her in this state. Mrs. Westen complained to Shauna that she was in a "lot of pain." Shauna asked her where her pain was and instead of pointing to her upper right quadrant she pointed to her head. Shauna was a nurse so she performed a quick neuro check and discovered a definite right-sided weakness. A brain scan was ordered which confirmed she had a ruptured vessel on the left side of her brain. She had suffered a stroke. As the ruptured vessel in her head continued to bleed the increasing intracranial pressure was the source of the increasing intensity of her headaches. Neglecting to determine the source of Mrs. Westen's pain had its long-term effects. Mrs. Westen recovered quickly from her gallbladder surgery but the recovery from her stroke was a slow tedious process including having to learn to read again.

Aside from physical pain, many patients suffer spiritual pain. Unfortunately nurses do not have clever, tangible tools to assess spiritual pain. Even if such tools existed, these plastic devices would only reveal "yes, my pain is pretty bad" and that is only part of the story. I wonder how many times we neglect to explore the source of someone's spiritual pain. Knowing the source of the spiritual distress, just as in knowing the source of physical pain, enables us to provide the care and resources to help ease the pain. Like the brain scan that identified the source of the patient's pain, we too can enlist outside resources. We can share Jesus as the source of peace and comfort to the soul. Jesus says, "Come to me, you who are tired and worried, and I will give you rest. Work with me and learn from me, for I am gentle and kind, and you will discover a biding peace in your soul. My requirements are easy and the load you carry will be light."[1] Jesus gives the criteria for assessing a spiritual need ("tired and worried") and also prescribes the remedy ("come unto me").

Bonnie Hunt

How Will I Know I'm Hurting?

The pager came to life and beeped its obnoxious little alarm until I pushed the button. The phone number flashed on the screen and I immediately recognized it as Mrs. Ryan's number. She was a long-term home health patient who continually experienced a variety of health problems that kept her as a "frequent flier" for the home health agency where I practiced as a RN. This was my weekend to be on-call and respond to any problems or emergencies that occurred. Mrs. Ryan's main problem was loneliness and she seemed to have an emergency every weekend.

I knew her well as I had cared for her for quite a while. Dialing her number, I wondered what might be the problem this time. After several rings, Mrs. Ryan answered the phone.

"Hello?"

"Mrs. Ryan, this is Nettie from the home health agency. Did you call?"

"Hello, Nettie. How are you?"

"I'm fine. How are you?" I answered politely. Wanting to get to the immediate problem, I continued, "Did you call, Mrs. Ryan? I had a page to call you."

"Oh, Nettie, yes, I called. Ohhh, Ohh, it's my right knee! Ohhh, it hurts sooooo bad!"

Mrs. Ryan moaned and groaned for added effect.

"Did you fall or injure your knee?"

"No, noooo, it just started hurting, ohhhh, ohhhh!"

"When did it start hurting?"

"Twenty years ago, Nettie." Mrs. Ryan answered quite seriously.

Knowing the patient had osteoarthritis for years, I knew she misunderstood my question.

Inspiration PRN: Stories About Nurses

She recently had a total knee replacement and was getting physical therapy through the home health agency.

"I mean when did it start hurting *today*?"

"This morning, Nettie. It just started aching. I think a cold front is coming in."

I asked a few more questions to assess her pain. Knowing her physician prescribed her pain medication while she was rehabilitating, I asked her if she had taken her pain medication.

"My pain medication? You think I should take my pain killers?"

"Yes, if you are in pain, take your pain medication."

"But, Nettie, how will I know I am hurting?"

Sounds silly doesn't it? Yet, how often do we have this attitude when we experience emotional pain in our lives? We continue to keep the pain alive. Do you ever relive over and over again situations in which you were hurt? Do you hold grudges when someone treated you wrongly? Sometimes we tend to keep the "hurting" going by harboring bad feelings toward those who harm us. It is quite human to be hurt when someone mistreats or takes advantage of us. It is natural to want to seek vengeance. Many times we allow the most insignificant occurrences to hurt us and become painful. Often it leads to hurting relationships with others. Yet it results in allowing the pain to manage our lives instead of us managing the pain in our lives. God has designed something to relieve pain in our lives: forgiveness. Forgiveness is the analgesic of choice for interpersonal bumps and bruises.

Our Savior showed us this during His life on earth. He knows our lives will be fuller and more fulfilling when we learn to manage the pain in our lives and depend on Him. He forgave even though falsehoods, rumors, and abuse were aimed at Him and His followers. He taught us to include forgiveness in our prayers. He told parables that taught forgiveness. Our Lord endured and suffered far more than any of us and forgave. We live because of His sacrifice and His forgiveness of our sins. Our very hope for eternity is based on the grace and yes, forgiveness He extends to us.

"If we confess our sins, He is faithful and just to forgive us our sins and to cleanse us from all unrighteousness."[1]

David Gerstle

Painful Confusion

"Honey, will you go over to Aunt Sue's and get some eggs? I need them to bake a cake today," she mumbled.

This is how I was greeted the morning I was assigned to Mrs. Sullivan on the orthopedic unit. She had fallen and broken her hip resulting in surgery three days ago. Since I worked on the PRN pool, the unit nurses gave me a little more history on Mrs. Sullivan's postoperative progress. About a day after surgery the patient became confused and was definitely not oriented to time and place. She wasn't doing well with sitting in a chair or working with the physical therapist. For whatever logic leading to these types of decisions, the nurses decided the Demerol injections were making her confused and they were just giving her Tylenol Extra Strength orally. They had decided since she was elderly that it would take a few days for the Demerol to "get out of her system" and then her confusion would clear up. Silently I wondered if her pain would "clear up" too.

"Honey, help me with the breakfast dishes now; I have lots to do today." Mrs. Sullivan continued.

"Good morning, Mrs. Sullivan. How are you today?" I greeted the small elderly woman.

Her silver hair was unkempt and sticking out in a variety of tangles and squirrels' nests. Her bed covers were twisted and rumpled as evidence of a nightlong battle against the wrist restraints applied to keep her from falling out of bed. Her eyes didn't quite focus on me and she didn't respond to my greeting. She certainly presented as an elderly woman living in the past without little to any relationship to reality.

I bent closer to her face and said, "I am your nurse today. How are you feeling?"

Inspiration PRN: Stories About Nurses

"What?"

Hey, a response. I repeated what I had said.

"My nurse? You are William. Quit this foolishness and go do your chores."

"Do you know where you are?"

"What?"

"Do you know where you are?"

"Hand me those canned peaches over there." Mrs. Sullivan pointed toward the corner of the room.

Realizing now that I wouldn't be documenting "Oriented X 3", I continued to make my assessment in between getting eggs and assisting making a peach cobbler. Upon assessing her affected hip, I found that just moving her leg elicited a painful response from Mrs. Sullivan.

"Ooooooooh! That's sore, don't do that."

It was obvious the patient was suffering and needed more analgesia than what Tylenol Extra Strength could provide. I left the room and checked her medication record. Indeed, the nurses were only giving Tylenol since the second evening after her surgery. This was just not enough for hip surgery, especially since physical therapy was an early part of recovery. Although I am not a fan of Demerol especially for the elderly, it was better than what Mrs. Sullivan had been receiving. Seeing that it was still ordered, I drew up the injection and returned to give it to Mrs. Sullivan. Some self-doubt entered my mind that this would sedate her too much for PT as well as truly increase her confusion. Checking the restraints and side rails, I left the room and checked my other patients.

Returning to Mrs. Sullivan's room, I found one of the nurse assistants feeding her breakfast. The patient was not cooperating very well and talking again about going to Aunt Sue's and all the chores needing to be done. Seeing the frustration on the assistant's face, I offered to finish feeding Mrs. Sullivan if she would return and bathe her in a little while and then help me get her in a chair. The nurse assistant made some comment about that was going to be a lot of fun and left the room. I continued to offer bites of oatmeal and promising Mrs. Sullivan that I would go to town right after breakfast and get a bag of sugar.

Late that morning the nurse assistant completed Mrs. Sullivan's bath and was ready to help me get her up in a chair. The move to the chair wasn't too bad since Mrs. Sullivan was a small patient and I a big nurse. Placing a sheet restraint around her, I asked her if she was having any pain.

"What?" she mumbled.

"I wonder if she can't hear," I remarked to the nurse assistant.

"I know I have to yell to make her hear me. I'll look in her table for a hearing aid," the assistant said as she began her search.

"Hey, here are her hearing aids and her glasses. In fact, here are her teeth."

"Good! We have the technology and know-how to rebuild her." I said as I reached for the hearing aids and placed them in Mrs. Sullivan's ears.

"Are you having any pain?"

"Any what?"

Turning to the assistant, "Hand me her glasses. We're not done yet."

Placing her glasses on her face, I repeated my question.

Looking at my face, Mrs. Sullivan mumbled, "My hip is sore. You know I fell on it the other day."

Interesting response. No more going to Aunt Sue's for eggs.

With a grin on her face the nurse assistant hands me freshly cleaned dentures, "The transformation can now be complete."

With the dentures now in place, I asked Mrs. Sullivan about her pain again.

With a tender and clear voice, she said, "My hip is sore but it is much better."

Reorienting her to place and time, Mrs. Sullivan carried on a rational conversation with me as I sat talking to her. She had a smile on her face and held my hand as we enjoyed this moment of lucidity.

The nurse assistant was intrigued with the change in Mrs. Sullivan.

"What did you do to make her so clear? She is like a new person."

"Well, I gave her some pain medication that worked. You know severe pain can cause confusion too."

"She is so sweet. I need to fix her up."

The nurse assistant asked Mrs. Sullivan if she could brush her hair.

"Of course, dear. I would like that."

I left the room as the "girls" enjoyed themselves with the makeover. Word got around the unit that the "male nurse from the pool" gave a Demerol injection to Mrs. Sullivan and cleared up her mental status. The physical therapist was thankful as it improved the patient's progress. The surgeon was happy since he could carry on a rational conversation with the patient. The nurses were skeptical at first but couldn't deny the improvement of Mrs. Sullivan. Hopefully, they rethought their pain management strategies. Best of all, Mrs. Sullivan was relieved of the severe pain and was quite happy for all the attention she was now getting.

Life can bring pain to all of us. The longer we have pain, the more severe it becomes. Many times with emotional and spiritual pain as with physical pain, we become confused and seek out ways to deal with the pain that are not effective. We may dwell on the pain and do nothing to relieve it, thus making it worse. We may try to deny the pain and suffer inside. We may try to cover up

Inspiration PRN: Stories About Nurses

the pain and act inappropriately thus affecting our relationships with others and with God. This results in even greater pain. God invites us to bring our burdens and trials and pain to Him. He promises to bear our burdens for us. He doesn't promise that we will never have pain, but He does promise He will never leave us to suffer alone. Don't let this world of pain confuse you and lead from the One who can provide comfort.

"Cast your burden on the Lord, and He shall sustain you; He shall never permit the righteous to be moved."[1]

David Gerstle

Solving the Wrong Problem

Orthopedic surgery patients share one thing in common—pain. Ben just underwent a lumbar laminectomy the day before and had complained of back pain throughout the night shift. The nurse caring for him during the night had medicated Ben for pain a couple of times throughout the shift. This was in addition to the analgesic dosages being delivered continuously through the PCA pump.

"He has not been able to get comfortable tonight and has not slept much. The pain is decreased when Ben is on his side, but never enough to get some decent sleep"; the nurse reported, "I don't know what else to do for him, so I am leaving him with you guys on the day shift."

Back surgery patients require a lot of pain medication after surgery. It is usually effective and allows for comfort and sleep. However, Ben was not finding this relief. The first thing nurses typically do is to check the PCA pump and ascertain that it is set for the proper dosages and that it is working properly. Sometimes additional analgesics must be given to relieve pain. The second thing typically done is to turn the patient and try position the patient for comfort. These interventions seemed to fail for Ben. It was now up to me to resolve the pain.

Greeting the patient, I began assessing him and hopefully discover why his pain was not being relieved.

"Man, my back has been killing me all night." Ben informed me as I talked to him.

Turning him on his side, I assessed his surgical dressing and noticed that the IV tubing from the PCA pump was stuck to the dressing. Upon further investigation, not only was it found to be stuck, but also it was taped down to the dressing. I had seen many dressings before, but I can't say I had ever seen such a technique before. I began peeling back the tape from the tubing and detaching it from the dressing. I began tugging on the last piece of tape from the lower part of the tubing when Ben began to cry out, "Ouch, that really hurts!"

"Sorry, the IV tubing is stuck to your dressing."

Removing the last piece of tape revealed that the edge of the connector on the extension tubing was gouging into Ben's skin next to the incision site. The connector left a fairly deep red impression where it had been pressed down by the tape and the weight of Ben's body.

"Hey, what did you do? My back feels better all of a sudden." The patient exclaimed.

"Well, Ben, I removed the proverbial 'thorn from your side'; it looks like we have been trying to solve the wrong problem."

It seems that we do this often in life. We suffer from problems, but don't recognize the cause. We look for sophisticated and complicated solutions to the wrong problems. Sometimes we don't want to acknowledge the real problem, so we attempt to deal with everything but what we need to deal with. Let God lead you in revealing problems to you and then ask for His help in coping with them.

"Deal bountifully with Your servant, that I may live and keep Your word. Open my eyes that I may see wondrous things from Your law."[1]

David Gerstle

A Shoulder to Cry On

It was early morning as I walked through the hospital hallways. This was the first of four days I was scheduled to work on the renal unit. As I approached the bank of elevators, I saw a man in his twenties. He was resting his head on the wall and sobbing.

"Sir, may I help you?" I asked.

Looking slowly at me, he barely whispers "My dad just died."

"May I call someone for you?"

"No, no, I'm OK" he said as he walked away from me and down the hall.

Twelve-year-old Laura was admitted for alcohol overdose. She and her friends opened her parent's liquor cabinet and began sampling its contents. Laura sampled far more than she could handle, became extremely intoxicated and passed out. She woke up in the emergency department with IVs running in her arms with her mother by her side. The nurse prepared the nasogastric tube to insert in her stomach and remove its contents. Laura was not having a good day and it wasn't likely to improve.

She was moved to the pediatric floor and the next day her mother decided to make an example of her daughter. She brought Laura's friends with her to her daughter's room.

Circling them around the bed, the mother began her tour of the IV running in Laura's arm, the tube running down her nose and the suction machine's hissing noises with the green bile vacillating up and down the tube. She pointed to Laura's pale face with petechiae around her bloodshot eyes and described in cruel detail how Laura vomited and retched while the tube was inserted down her nose. She mentioned several

Inspiration PRN: Stories About Nurses

times how her stomach was pumped and how vile the smell of vomit was in the air. Her mother made the point several times that only stupid kids drink. A single tear sliding down Laura's cheek was the only sign of how much her mother's words stung.

Amy works as a nurse on the orthopedic unit. During report, the unit secretary tells her she has an emergency phone call. She takes the call at the desk and listens for a few minutes. Suddenly, she cries out, "No, no, no!" and throws the telephone to the floor. She drops to a chair, lays her head on the counter, and weeps uncontrollably. She just found out that her two-year-old grandson did not survive a severe asthma attack. The news devastates her.

This world has a lot of hurt in it. Nurses throughout their careers will interact with many people who experience trauma, pain, death, and loss. All of us at some point will experience pain of one type or another. It is difficult to handle it all alone. Although this world can be a dark hurtful place, God is still in control. As nurses, we can share God's strength to our patients by offering a shoulder to cry on, compassion, and support. We can express our faith that even when disastrous things occur in life, God still cares even when His presence seems far away. Always invite God to be in your nursing practice as you minister to your patients.

Davie Gerstle

Out of the Darkness

"Good morning, Jeremy." I said as I clicked on the lights.

A soft mumble came from the general direction of the bed. Jeremy had his head covered up with the sheet and blankets.

"Mind if I open the blinds?" I said as I stepped toward the window.

"Leave 'em closed." came the quiet almost indiscernible response from the form in the bed.

Deciding not to push the issue, I stepped away from the window.

"I tell you what, Jeremy. I will leave for now and let you wake up a little more. When I come back, we will get your morning started with breakfast."

Leaving the room, I thought that if I took it slowly, maybe Jeremy would talk to me about how he was feeling. It just wasn't like him to hide under the covers when someone came into his room. He was normally a very social kid.

Jeremy had been on the pediatric wing for several weeks now. The nursing staff had all become well acquainted with the well-mannered 10-year-old. A severe infection landed Jeremy in the hospital. He had gone swimming with his family in a river near their home and had stepped on a submerged branch with thorns. A sharp thorn had pierced the bottom of his foot leaving a portal for any bacteria from the thorn and river water to enter. Although first aid had been given to treat his wound, Jeremy succumbed to an infection. A large abscess had formed requiring surgery to incise and drain it. Unfortunately, the organisms causing the infection were resistant to a number of antibiotics thus leading to a non-healing wound. The physicians were trying to find antibiotics that would be effective against the invading bacteria. This all resulted in a long hospital stay and isolation due to the draining wound.

The nurses assigned to Jeremy were diligent in providing his physical care that involved trips to the whirlpool, dressing changes, and administering antibiotics. Other than trips to the whirlpool, strict contact isolation demanded that Jeremy remain in his room. He seemed to tolerate it well; the nurses kept up a good rapport with him and tried to make his days and nights as pleasant as possible. Although time was limited, some time was given to playing card games, computer games, and just good old-fashioned "goofing off."

The fourth week of hospitalization did not bring any further progress in wound healing. The physicians were becoming frustrated and were unsure as to what path to take next. The nurses became even more diligent in maintaining strict wound care and isolation. Much more attention was given to the physical care and as a result less attention was given to Jeremy's social and spiritual needs. Less time was given to play. Less time was spent with him in his isolation room as an effort to decrease his risk for getting secondary infections from the environment.

Slowly and subtly, Jeremy began to withdraw. He talked less and less with the nurses and physicians. He lost interest in playing games and slept more. The staff thought that he was just getting tired from the routine of the hospital and would soon "snap" out of it. But, Jeremy didn't "snap" out of it. He began requesting that the window blinds be kept closed. Next, he insisted that the room lights be turned out except when care was being given. Soon after, he stopped watching television and listening to the radio.

This had been going on for several days when I was assigned to care for Jeremy. I had cared for Jeremy many times before, but had not been assigned to him for a while since I was also a relief charge nurse. I walked into his darkened room after shift report that morning.

"Knock, knock. Breakfast is served, Your Majesty." I announced as I opened Jeremy's door.

The lights were again turned off and Jeremy's back was turned toward me. I set down the tray on the bedside table.

"Are you hungry, Jeremy?"

"No" he whispered, still with his back toward me.

I sat down on the chair next to the bed and just listened to the sounds in the room. Except for Jeremy's breathing and my own, there were no other sounds; no music, no television, not even any beeps from the IV pump. The lights were still off with the only illumination coming from around the closed blinds and the LED screen on the IV pump. This was the environment that Jeremy lived in and created by keeping everything dark and quiet. He had in essence "entombed" himself in his isolation. Was he trying to tell us something in this way that he could not tell us in words?

"Jeremy, how are you feeling today?"

No response.

"Jeremy, can you turn over and look at me?"

Again, no response.

I didn't know what to do, but I knew that Jeremy needed me to help him. So, with a silent prayer asking for guidance, I did nothing. I just sat there silently.

A few minutes passed and Jeremy turned over just enough to see if I was still there. Seeing me, he turned his back to me again. I stood up and placed my hand on his shoulder.

"Tell me what's wrong, Jeremy."

An eternally long pause occurred before I heard his trembling answer.

"I'm going to die."

Shocked, I asked, "Why do you think you are going to die?"

Crying, Jeremy explained that he had noticed that the nurses weren't spending as much time with him as they had done in the past because they had given up on him. He had also heard the physicians talking outside his door about how the antibiotics weren't working and that they didn't know what to do.

Keeping my hand on his shoulder to comfort him, I assured Jeremy that he wasn't going to die. I told him that the nurses were just spending more time on taking care of him so they didn't have as much time to spend doing fun things with him. I also told him that his doctors were going to find the right medication for him and that no one was giving up.

I left the room again to give Jeremy some time to cry and to share his feelings with the nurses and physicians.

Realizing that Jeremy was going into depression, we formed a plan of care to maintain his psychological, social, and spiritual well being. Of course the mandatory psychiatry consult was made, but even more important than that, we became diligent with spending time with Jeremy to do nothing more than to have fun - games, telling jokes, and "goofing off" as we were diligent with his wound care.

Since we could keep his wound covered for the trip to the whirlpool, we also kept it covered as we took him outside in the sunshine. In fact we made many such trips, often on our own time since a busy nursing unit doesn't allow for much latitude.

It all soon paid off; Jeremy returned to his easygoing social self. He once again loved the light and sunshine, music, games, and conversation. Believe it or not, Jeremy began to heal without any change in antibiotics. The bacteria count went down and the wound began to heal. Jeremy was soon discharged home as a boy who loved sunshine and people instead of a boy desiring darkness and silence.

Life can bring hardships that seem too heavy to bear. Many times, these hardships are not known by those around the one bearing them. Have you ever had the experience of carrying such a burden that you began to withdraw from your friends and family? Soon you see everything darkly and feel you must be alone in your misery. Yet, you never have to be alone. God is always there and invites you to call on Him. He does not promise that all of your burdens will be removed, but He does promise He will carry them for you.

"Take my yoke upon you and learn from Me, for I am gentle and lowly in heart and you will find rest for your souls. For My yoke is easy and My burden is light."[1]

David Gerstle

CCU Madness

"Where are my cigarettes?" demanded the myocardial infarction (MI) patient.

"Mr. Walker, you have just had a heart attack. We have put your cigarettes up with the rest of your belongings."

"I want them now!" he demanded.

The heart monitor was going wild as his anger became worse.

"You can't have them," the nurse protested. "You may have another heart attack if you smoke!"

I was a junior nursing student assigned to the CCU that day and was a witness to this drama unfolding before me. I am thinking to myself, this man is going to have a heart attack if he *doesn't* get a smoke! About that time, Mr. Walker begins to remove the cardiac monitor leads from his chest. He next pulls off his oxygen nasal cannula and then pulls out his IV. He has enough presence of mind to hold pressure on the IV site with his fingers.

Mr. Walker stomps out of his CCU room with his patient gown barely covering his ample body. He walks into the nurses' station and begins opening drawers looking for his cigarettes.

"Give me my cigarettes *NOW!*" he bellows. There was no mistake, and he was serious. Dead serious, perhaps literally, as mad as he was. His blood pressure had to be over the top.

Hearing all of the commotion and yelling, the nurse manager came around the corner to find out what was happening.

Mr. Walker was livid. "My cigarettes-*NOW!*" he hissed.

Inspiration PRN: Stories About Nurses

Seeing how upset this MI patient was, the manager pulls out his cigarettes and lighter from their hiding place and hands them to him. Mr. Walker grabs them and walks out of the CCU, not a bit concerned that the moon had risen in the back of his "I-see-you" patient gown.

The nurse manager spots me standing by the desk. "You! Go with him and don't let him out of your sight!"

I took a long hard swallow and headed through the CCU automatic doors. I actually thought to grab an extra gown for the patient as I passed the linen cart. Heading out the doors and down the hall, I mentally reviewed the steps of CPR. Let's see, first you shake the victim and establish unresponsiveness. Of course, with Mr. Walker, you must be sure to not get burned by the inevitable cigarette dangling from his lips.

As I walked toward the waiting room, there was Mr. Walker, sucking on a cigarette. He actually looked better than he did a moment ago screaming for his cigarettes. He even had a shadow of a smile on his face.

"What do you want?" he growled at me as I approached him. He knew why I was there.

Being a student, I wasn't sure what I should do. But I did know I shouldn't try to get his cigarettes from him. I doubt it would do much good to try and convince him to return to the CCU now- he was enjoying the nicotine too much. He needed it (this was before the patches). So I just sat down on a chair across from him, holding the extra gown. I didn't say a thing.

"You brought me a gown," he said quietly.

"Oh, yes, I though you might be cold" I replied.

Mr. Walker laughed, "Not to mention I am giving everybody a peep show."

"That too." I said. Then we just sat there quietly as Mr. Walker smoked. He dropped his ashes in his hand as he did.

After a while, Mr. Walker said, "I guess you want me to go back to the CCU."

"That would be the best thing for you."

"I suppose you want these," as he held up his cigarettes and lighter.

"They may not be helping your heart. I'm sure your doctor will help you with those."

"Yeah, I know." he sighed.

"I guess I made a real spectacle of myself in there. I was scared and smoking calms me down."

I simply nodded and told him it was ok. We walked slowly back to the CCU together. I helped him get back into bed and hooked him back up to the cardiac monitor and oxygen.

The nurse manger gave me a congratulatory pat on the back as she entered the room. She began to assess Mr. Walker for any damage done. As I turned to leave to check on my assigned patient, Mr. Walker grabbed my arm and said one word, "Thanks."

Thanks for what? I just sat with him while he smoked. I didn't use any persuasion techniques to talk him back into the CCU. I didn't scold him and tell him he was gambling with his life. I didn't lecture him on the evils of tobacco. I didn't judge him. I just sat there with him.

It then occurred to me that was why he thanked me. He knew he shouldn't have become so upset and demand his cigarettes. He knew he shouldn't smoke. He knew having a heart attack was serious. He just needed someone to be with him as he did a foolish thing.

Nurses get frustrated when they teach patients to do all of the right things and then they don't do it. Nurses are puzzled when patients do things that are bad for them. Yet, in spite of this, nurses don't abandon their patients when they don't comply.

Neither does God when we as sinners keep on sinning. He doesn't abandon us. He stays by our side while we do foolish things. What happens many times is we abandon God. We leave Him; He doesn't leave us. Sometimes we feel we aren't good enough to be accepted by God, and that we must deserve to be loved by Him. God is Love. He accepts us where we are. We must accept Him in our lives, then He will make us deserving through His covering of our sins with His Perfect Life. How do we do this? By inviting Him into our lives and know that He is God and is in control of all things. He never leaves us; He remains by our side.

"Create in me a clean heart, O God. And renew a steadfast spirit within me. Do not cast me away from Your presence. And do not take Your Holy Spirit from me."[1]

David Gerstle

Left to Die

A new year was just dawning as I walked into the hospital for my day shift on New Year's Day. I pondered what patients the typical New Year's Eve celebrating and indiscretions may bring to the medical unit on which I worked. I was hoping for a nice quiet day. My thoughts were interrupted as I entered the hall leading to the elevators when I heard, "Clear the hall! We're coming through!" "Watch out!"

I looked up to see three emergency room nurses racing with a gurney carrying a pale young man in cardiac arrest. One nurse was guiding the front of the gurney and squeezing the ambu bag and another was pushing from behind. The third nurse was straddled across the patient and administering chest compressions. Expressions of desperation were on the nurses' faces as they rushed down the hall toward the emergency room.

As they passed, I wondered why the patient wasn't brought in by ambulance and why they were coming from the direction of the old emergency room that had recently been closed when the new one was built on the other side of the hospital. In the days to come, I would know the answers to these questions.

A few days after this incident, I was working the evening shift. The charge nurse stopped in the hall and told me I was getting a transfer patient from the intensive care unit (ICU). She said the patient was on a ventilator, but was also a DNR (do not resuscitate) patient. Our unit was staffed with a respiratory therapist who assisted the nursing staff in monitoring patients on ventilators. However, it was a bit unusual to have a DNR patient on a ventilator. The ICU nurse would give me report when she got up there. I went to prepare the room and check on my other patients before the new arrival came. The respiratory therapist was already setting up the ventilator in the assigned room.

It wasn't long before the new patient arrived. He was attached to a cardiac monitor and IV pump. The patient was intubated and being "bagged" during the trip from the ICU to our nursing unit. Skillfully, all of us worked together to move the patient from the ICU bed to the bed in the room. The ventilator was quickly connected and the patient assessed. The ICU nurse began to give a report on the patient:

"This is a 22-year-old male who is brain dead post cardiac arrest. He was apparently partying on New Year's Eve and overdosed on dope and alcohol. He was found lying unconscious by a worker early New Year's Day at the old emergency room entrance. The worker called the emergency room and some staff went down there. The patient was in full arrest when they arrived. They resuscitated him, but brain damage had already occurred. He has a flat EEG times two and will be getting another one soon."

The rest of the report consisted of vital signs, assessment findings, medications, and IV fluid counts. Of course, I realized as soon as report began that this was the same patient that I saw being wheeled down the hall that New Year's morning. It was a horrible thought that this young man had lain dying on the sidewalk at the wrong end of the hospital. How did he get there? Where were his friends?

After the report, the ICU nurse said his mother had been staying with him around the clock, but the nursing staff had sent her home to get some much needed rest, but she was coming up to the floor this evening.

"How was the mother coping with all of this?" I asked.

"She is doing ok. She reads the Bible to him every day."

"Does she know how he wound up at the old emergency entrance?"

"We asked her that. Evidently, his friends (the nurse makes air quotation marks as she said this) dumped him out there. They didn't want to be questioned about their doping so they just left him there. One of them felt guilty so he told the mother what happened. They had been partying and passed around some pills after they were already drunk. The patient was quite intoxicated and took more dope than the others. The one who called the mother only drank and didn't take any. He was the one who thought to at least take him to the hospital. The others were going to just leave him where they were partying. They were more concerned about staying out of trouble."

"Wow, that is just plain cold-hearted."

"Yes, just another example of our fine upstanding citizens," the ICU nurse said sarcastically as she departed.

Later that evening, the mother came to her son's room. She had not told anyone she had arrived. As I entered the room to check on the patient, I found Mom reading the Bible out loud to her son. I introduced myself and not wanting to interrupt any further quietly left the room. Over the next couple of days, the mother kept vigilance over her son. We began to build rapport and she shared with me her faith in God and her love for her son.

"My boy was always a handful as he grew up. He chose friends who were not going down the right road, so I would always tell him I was praying for him and that I loved him. I am still praying for him and I will never give up on him. I want my boy to live, but he is in God's Hands now."

Each day when the mother would have to leave to check on things at home, she would come by the nurses' station and ask me to watch over her son while she was gone. As I checked on him after she left, I noticed she would leave her Bible open to Psalm 23 on the bedside table. Her faith was never wavering and her devotion to her son never waning.

The third shift that I cared for this mother's son was the day he died. I had just returned from supper break when the nurse who was covering for me told me his heart had stopped just moments before. We entered his room and saw that he had expired. There were no signs of life as the ventilator continued to force air into his lungs. The mother had just gone home for a while, so I called her to return to the hospital. Without saying it, she knew her son was gone. When the mother returned, the physician on call came to the floor, pronounced the patient's death, and shut off the ventilator. With tears in her eyes, she thanked everyone for the care her son had received.

"I loved my son and I never gave up on him. He was my boy. Although he did not survive, I have faith in God. My son is still in His Hands now."

The mother's son was left for dead that early New Year's morning. His "friends" threw him out on the sidewalk like so much garbage. They were more concerned about themselves than whether this young man lived or died. They were not friends that stuck with him in a time of need. They did not value his life. Yet, his mother did not give up on him. Although there was nothing she could do and the outcome inevitable, she never abandoned him, never gave up praying for him. God does not give up on us even though sometimes it feels that way. He doesn't throw us away when we falter or choose another path. He doesn't turn His back to us when we fail. In bad times God doesn't walk away from us, He walks with us. He sticks closer than a brother.

"A man of many companions may come to ruin, but there is a friend who sticks closer than a brother."[1]

David Gerstle

The Way Home

Food, Fun, Forum! A catchy title? I thought so. Every so often the nursing faculty wanted to have the different levels of nursing students come together to clarify some expectations such as, their upcoming summer practicum or graduation requirements or provide information regarding NCLEX (the national licensing exam) and to encourage any questions or suggestions the students might have. The catchy title worked! The sessions were well attended with both faculty and students benefitting from the forum. They also enjoyed mingling over food and would have a good laugh together over a skit or video presentation from upperclassmen. Needless to say, much valuable feedback comes from these sessions which help the faculty understand some of the students' problems as well as the students feeling they were making a positive contribution to the program.

As usual, at the end of one such session, the moderator was encouraging suggestions or questions when a hand shot up from the back row. "You give us excellent directions how to get to our clinicals, but you don't tell us how get back," lamented a fundamentals student. Chuckling, I thought to myself, "Well! Just go back the way you came." I am glad I did not make that comment out loud. Because on second thought I realized that in the metropolitan area where the majority of the clinical sites were located are one-way streets. Traveling to the clinical area would take you one way but when returning from the clinical area was a different story. Exiting the clinical area required a quick maneuver to the far left-hand lane of a four-lane road. Then one would have to cut though a residential street to another main thoroughfare going one way in the direction back to school. However, this thoroughfare dead ended into another major road so a left-hand turn was required and then in a few blocks one would have to ease right to take you back to the road that you came on and from then on it was the same way you came. As silly as it sounded at first, it was a legitimate comment.

If we pray as King David did "Lord...Help me know your way and give me strength to follow it and do what is right" (Psalm 5:8), keep in mind that God never entertains the notion that when we ask for directions that our comments are silly. For He promises that He will "lead (us) along roads (we) have not known and guide (us) along paths that are new...He will turn darkness into light and make the rough spots smooth...and not forsake us."[1]

When asking God directions, here is a sobering thought. "The Lords says, "My thoughts are not your thoughts, neither are my ways your ways"...but the good news is "As the heavens are higher than the earth, so are My thoughts higher than your thoughts and My ways higher than your ways."[2] Probably the most comforting promise of all when needing directions is found in that most familiar Psalms. Psalms 23 tells us that he leads us beside quiet waters, walks with us through a valley of frightful shadows when facing death...His rod and staff protect us...His goodness and mercy will be with us every day of our lives.

God bids us to daily ask for instructions "So make God's kingdom and His righteousness first in your life, and all the other things will be given to you as you need them."[2] These "other things" include the promise in Isaiah. "If you start turning to the right or to the left you will hear a still, small voice telling you, 'Over here is the way to walk'."[3] Now that is the best way (route?) home!

Bonnie Hunt

Plans

Craig had been planning a career in anesthesia for several years. He had even moved from the "comforts of home" to a large strange city to work in intensive care units in the hospital where the school of anesthesia of his choice was located.

After working for several years, he applied to the school of anesthesia. His interview with the faculty was a very positive experience and he felt fairly confident he would be one of the four candidates that would be accepted. This confidence did not last long for in a few weeks he suffered the disappointment of not being admitted to the program. His blighted hope was somewhat lessened by the conviction that God was still leading in the direction of anesthesia and the fact that the faculty had told him he would be a priority candidate when he reapplied next year. So he continued to work in an intensive care unit eagerly anticipating the next spring when he would be admitted to the anesthesia program.

In May of the next year the "acceptances" were sent out. Craig could not believe his eyes as he read that he had been placed on the "alternate" list. Being "first" alternate did not diminish his devastating disappointment. Being his mother, I felt his keen disappointment. As we talked on the phone, I was searching for something comforting to say. "Maybe one of the candidates will have to drop out before next fall," I suggested trying to sound optimistic. "Well! That is very unlikely since it is so difficult to be admitted in anesthesia these days," he groaned. Before hanging up I promised Craig that I would continue to pray for him and his career choice and that the Lord would give him peace of mind and wisdom for the future. Even though

Inspiration PRN: Stories About Nurses

somewhat disillusioned he said he had already committed his situation to the Lord and asked for guidance.

Upon returning from my vacation in early June, the first words that greeted me from Craig's older brother, who lived with me at the time, was "Craig got into anesthesia school!" Unbeknown to Craig or the faculty, one of the candidates had applied to two schools of anesthesia. Shortly after I left for vacation, this candidate notified the school of anesthesia where Craig had applied that he had been accepted in another school and wanted to withdraw his name as a candidate. Now Craig, being the first alternate could take his place.

When Craig called to discuss the quick change in events he humbly confessed, "Even though my faith that God was leading in my life never wavered, this experience has taught me a valuable lesson." Then Craig mused, "'The best laid plans of mice and men' can go afoul and the future at times can appear pretty dismal but God is still in charge."

"Commit your way unto the Lord; trust also in Him; and he shall bring it to pass."[1] "Delight thyself also in the Lord; and he shall give you the desires of your heart."[2]

Isn't there a lesson here for all of us?

Bonnie Hunt

"O DEATH, WHERE IS THY STING?"

"Though I walk through the valley of the shadow of death..."

The patient was gasping for breath and clutching his chest with his eyes rolled toward the back of his head...members of his family standing by his bedside were ringing their hands and not so quietly sobbing...and I, the student nurse, sent to observe someone dying was standing close by wondering why someone or something couldn't be done to help this pitiful soul. When the gasping subsided and the patient went limp, the family wailed all the louder. I slipped out of the room having no idea of what to do since I had only been hustled in to witness death-taking place.

This was in the days before CPR and the concept of letting one die with dignity. When I asked what caused the man's death, I thought they said something about his heart; but I don't really remember for sure. But I do remember that, unfortunately, this experience formed my image of how one goes about the process of dying. It left me confused about the notion that when one dies they just "fall asleep in Jesus."

Even at forty, she was too young to be dying of colon cancer. I am not sure how long the battle against this monster of a disease had been, but my first encounter with Marlene was a few days after she had been admitted to the hospital for the last agonizing days of her life. I don't know why I used the word "agonizing" to describe her last days...I guess I used that word because it was agonizing for the family and me. Actually, Marlene was quite at peace with the experience. It was the peaceful expression on her face that always caught me off guard as she lay quietly in bed with her hands folded over her chest. As I performed the daily assessment, I would ask was there anything I could do for her. Sometimes she would ask to be turned or request a sip of water or would just give a weak smile and say she was "all right for now."

Since I worked the evening shift her husband would fill me in on what kind of day she had and then before leaving the room I would pat her arm and tell her I would check on her frequently. One evening as I was preparing to leave her room, she opened her eyes and looked up at me and said, "I like your wig." I smiled and whispered, "It's not a wig it's my real hair." She responded "That's o.k. I have one just like it at home." I marveled to my self this woman is dying and she has the strength to comment on my hair. Wow! The very next evening after doing her assessment, it seemed to me she would not last though the night. She was so weak she could barely open her eyes to acknowledge my presence. I checked on her and her husband more frequently that evening feeling for sure that would be the last time I would see them.

To my surprise when I arrived the next evening I saw that Marlene was still in her room. I quietly entered finding her respirations were shallow and weak and she seemed to be hanging on "by a thread" as the expression goes. Taking her wrist to feel for a pulse, she opened her eyes looked up at me and weakly but quite audibly said, "I fooled you, I'm still here." I couldn't help but smile and think "wow" again, this woman still has a sense of humor. I was off the next day and the nurse that took care of her during the night said that she just quietly "slipped away" in the early morning. It amazed me how Marlene had accepted her immortality in such a quiet, unassuming way, so unlike the experience I witnessed as a student.

Even though I went off to graduate school and focused on oncology nursing I never ceased to be surprised how my patients dealt with the process of death and dying, again so unlike the experience I had as a student. One time I walked in a room to check on a dying patient and found the patient telling her husband where to look in the closet for the outfit she wanted to be buried in. I went away wondering how one could make such plans as life is ebbing away. One wife just a few weeks before her death made a prioritized list of women for her husband to consider marrying after she died. She was suffering with pancreatic cancer and knew her death would not be easy. I puzzled over how could she be worrying about her husband's welfare at a time like this.

Another time I entered a patient's room to find eight people crammed around the bedside of this dying relative. Mostly they were talking among themselves but occasionally would include the patient by asking if she remembered so and so or ask her a question. Even though very weak the patient would try to respond. As I did my assessment, I sensed all these people were making her anxious. I asked her if she wanted them to leave the room for a while. She nodded "no." A few minutes later I had to hang some IV fluids and I continued to sense she was anxious so I asked her again if she would like for her family to leave the room, this time she nodded "yes." The family all got up, left the room but stood around in the hall by her door. I followed them out. About three or four minutes later I noticed one of the relatives with a bewildered look on her face peeking in the room. I went back into the room and checked on the patient. She had died. The relative that had been peeking in the room looked at me in astonishment and said, "She wanted us out so she could die in peace, didn't she?" And that was the way it seemed, with every one out of the room she could relax and let go peacefully.

My concept of how one goes about the process of dying was rapidly changing. What I observed was that all these patients had come to grips with the inevitable. Death and dying, like birthing, are part of the cycle of

Inspiration PRN: Stories About Nurses

life. What gave them acceptance was their belief in God and his promise that truly "The Lord is my shepherd I will lack nothing. He lets me lie down in green pastures. He leads me beside quiet water. He restores the strength of my soul. He guides me along paths of righteousness. Even when I have to walk through a valley of frightful shadows facing death, I will fear no evil, because you are with me. Your rod and staff protect me. Your goodness and mercy will be with me every day of my life, and I will live with you in your house forever."

Evidence of their faith was seen in the spiritual artifacts around their room as well as patient, family members and me sharing our favorite texts with each other, which most often in these circumstances was the 23rd Psalm.

For over a year she battled throat cancer. Numerous surgeries, chemotherapy, and radiation still had not conquered the malignancy. Mrs. Ryan was admitted to the hospital since her family could no longer care for her at home. The pain and all of the needs of a patient confined to bed became overwhelming for them. They were a close-knit family and were faithful in visiting her each day in the hospital. Although they could no longer take care of her physical need, they were there to meet her other needs.

One night, Mrs. Ryan's condition worsened. She was having difficulty breathing and did not respond when spoken too. The night nurse called the family and told them that Mrs. Ryan was not doing well and that they should come to the hospital. Late at night, her family gathered around her bed. The nurse passed out hymnals borrowed from the hospital chapel so they could sing to Mrs. Ryan some of her favorite hymns. As the family sang late into the night, Mrs. Ryan's breathing eased, she became more alert and looked around the room. Sensing she was doing better now the family left for home.

During the morning nurses' report, the night nurse related how Mrs. Ryan seemed to be dying, but then improved after her family arrived. After report, I went into her room.

Mrs. Ryan was awake.

"How are you doing this morning?" I asked.

"I think I disappointed my family last night," she replied.

Afraid she may be distressed about the night's events, I asked, "What do you mean?"

"Well, I was having a little trouble breathing and the nurse became concerned. The next thing I knew, my family is around my bed singing hymns. I think I was supposed to die last night and I didn't do it." She then laughed and said, "The singing helped me sleep, and maybe that's why I recovered!"

Mrs. Ryan was a Christian and her assurance of eternal life was intact. Death was not a frightening thing to her. She found humor in the "hymn-fest."

About two weeks later, Mrs. Ryan did lose her battle to cancer. It happened at night and yes, while her family surrounded her bed singing from the hymnals the nurse had borrowed. This time she did not awaken, but had the assurance she will awaken again and meet her Savior at the Second Coming.

Mrs. Ryan's comfort and acceptance when facing the inevitable is described in Proverbs "...but even in death, the HOPE of the righteous is their refuge."[1] That hope is "...but all who believe in Christ will be changed and live forever. In a moment, in the blink of an eye, God will change us. When the trumpet sounds, the dead will be resurrected, those who are still living will be transformed and all of us will be given glorious bodies that will never die."[2]

David Gerstle & Bonnie Hunt

A New Beginning

Air abruptly filled her lungs and her mind began to clear. Becoming more aware, she realized that she was in a grave. Being only five feet and four inches tall, she could only see the sides of the grave. Looking toward her feet, she saw that she was standing in an opened casket. This is her grave! Looking upward, she saw that the sky was bright and filled with heavenly beings. Angels? In the center of all this was another being sitting on a throne in the midst of a huge and glorious cloud. He had a crown and scepter emanating a great and awesome light. God?

Only moments passed when an angel hovered above her grave. She felt that she knew him; his presence seemed familiar. Was he her guardian angel? Before she knew what was happening, she was no longer in the grave, but was holding the angel's hand and flying toward the clouds. She wasn't afraid as they rose above the earth with the other celestial beings. Numerous other angels filled the skies leading their charges to the heavens above. Was this a dream? Was it really happening? She wasn't sure, as it seemed so real. She had believed since she was a little girl that Jesus would come again and take His followers to heaven. She had been afraid of death, but now felt calm.

Glancing to her left, she saw someone she knew. Someone who cared for her. Tina? It couldn't be! Then her memory rushed into her mind. The last thing she recalled before she found herself standing in her own grave was that she could not breathe and was fighting for her life. Tina, her nurse was with her. She remembered now that she was in the intensive care unit. She had been in a car accident and had severely fractured her left leg[**]. The orthopedic surgeon had to insert a Steinman

---

[**] The medical events and details are based on an actual patient.

pin and place her in traction. Before going to the ICU, she had been on the orthopedic unit and had difficulty breathing. She had undergone a lung scan that revealed fat emboli in her pulmonary vessels. Her doctors had told her and her parents that this was very serious. She was only 17 and this news petrified her with fear.

Her nurse, Tina, was diligent in caring for her and assessing her for any distress and changes in her vital signs. Tina spent time with her, giving words of encouragement and comfort. She held her hand and talked to her as she went about her work. Tina was a caring and thoughtful nurse as well as a consummate expert in critical care. Her young patient depended on her for her very survival.

The young patient had more and more difficulty breathing when the alarms on the monitor went off. Tina was by her side and began emergency procedures immediately. The other nurses and physician went into action in a desperate attempt to reverse the failure of her vital functions. Yet, the emboli's devastating effects on the pulmonary circulation were too much to counteract with even the most aggressive treatment. Her body was starving for oxygen. She was losing the fight. Tina let the others manage the code as she held her hand. The nurse looked into her eyes and saw the fear losing its grip as she slipped into unconsciousness, then death. The last thing the young girl saw was the compassion in the nurse's eyes.

Nurses may see death frequently throughout their careers; which can be especially discouraging when the patients are young. It is a helpless feeling when trying to stop death. Nurses want to make people "better." When death occurs it seems as the epitome of failure and their efforts appear futile. Yet, easing patients' and their families' fears and pain in the event of death are an important aspect of nursing care. Helping patients in this most desperate time has great impact not only on the ones dying, but on their loved ones as well. In fact, it may have an everlasting impact.

God gets blamed for a lot of things including death. Yet He never intended for death to occur. Sin entered this world and led to death in all of God's creation. Showing compassion and genuine caring may influence others' picture of God, particularly when death occurs. Providing comfort and dignity is also paramount. Nurses' presence and interventions cannot be more important. Take courage, nurses, and know that your care for a dying patient is not the end, but a new beginning.

"Let not your heart be troubled, you believe in God, believe also in me. In My Father's house are many mansions; if it were not so, I would have told you, I go to prepare a place for you. And if I go and prepare a place for you, I will come again and receive you to Myself that where I am, there you may be also."[1]

David Gerstle

Will to Live, Will to Die

Mrs. Clark's back had been hurting her for months when she finally decided to go to the doctor. After examining her, Mrs. Clark's family physician referred her to an orthopedic surgeon for further evaluation. A CT Scan showed a mass on the spine and a myelogram confirmed that a herniated disc was the cause of the back pain. A lumbar laminectomy and fusion were subsequently scheduled to surgically correct the defect. Mrs. Clark was assured by the surgeon and the nursing staff that this type of surgery was effective and as routine as any other surgery and that the pain she had been experiencing would be relieved as she recovered from the surgery. She was given instructions on what to expect after surgery- IVs, ambulation, pain control, wearing back support corsets. She was prepared for surgery and off she went to the OR for the "routine" back surgery everyone expected. However, the surgery and subsequent occurrences after surgery were anything but routine.

Upon exposing the surgical site and visualizing the "herniated disc," the surgeon recognized that the tissue was abnormal. A specimen was taken and sent to the pathologist for identification and cytology examination. It was soon known that the mass was a tumor that was inoperable and held further suffering and ultimately death for the patient. Further testing would need to be done to confirm the type of malignancy and determine if there was any type of treatment available to treat it. For now the surgeon could only close the incision.

The next morning the surgeon told Mrs. Clark what they had found and that it was not yet known if there was anything that could be done at this point. Although a strong woman, Mrs. Clark cried and shared with the surgeon and her nurse that morning that she had no family except a niece who had a drug problem and was always coming around asking for money. She voiced her concern that there was no one who could care for her as her condition worsened. She was afraid that her niece would take advantage of her in this state and steal from her to support her drug habit. Her future looked very bleak to her.

Mrs. Clark spent the next several days in the hospital recovering from her surgery. I was assigned to care for her during this period of time. Her worst fears of her niece discovering that she was ill were realized as one day the niece and her boyfriend showed up at the hospital. They of course asked for money and seeing that she was not able to care for herself, they told Mrs. Clark that maybe they should stay at her house. Mrs. Clark feared that this was just an excuse to get into her house so they could take anything of value and sell it. Of course she refused to let them have the keys and after they left, she shared with me that she was afraid that they would continue to come around and try to get money from her as well as break into her house. She stated that she just didn't want to live out the rest of her days fearing what her niece would do.

"I would just as soon die now than to worry all the time about her taking advantage of me," she said.

After this visit, Mrs. Clark could not walk as well as she did before and seemed to have greater pain. Morphine did not seem to have the same analgesic effect as it had before. When I brought in another injection of the pain medication, Mrs. Clark would ask me, "Can't you just give me a little more than what I should get? You know what I mean, so I won't breathe any more." "I really have no reason to live any longer; just give me too much; no one will ever know."

She would request the same thing the next day and the next. I notified the physician to let him know and that I was quite concerned about her despondency.

Couldn't we do something about this niece who was making a bad situation worse for this patient with inoperable cancer? It was agreed that we needed to intervene. We notified the social worker and the physician made a referral to a psychologist to visit Mrs. Clark I felt better that we had taken some steps to help her deal with this complicated situation. However, none of these interventions were ever to occur.

I entered Mrs. Clark's room early the next day; right after report. Nothing eventful had been noted during the night, but Mrs. Clark looked different to me. She seemed very sad, yet resolved about what I didn't know. I asked her if she had any pain. She replied that it was no more than usual. As was our routine every morning, I helped her put on her back support corset so she could sit up for breakfast. As I helped her to her feet, she stood for a moment and then said it hurt too much and she wanted to lie back down. I eased her back onto the bed and loosened her corset.

"My chest hurts" she said.

I took her vital signs and all was normal, but she was now perspiring and pale. I immediately called the physician who ordered a STAT EKG. He came to the floor shortly thereafter. Looking at the EKG, he noted that it was normal. We both went into the patient's room. Clinically nothing had changed. He asked me to give a dose of pain medication to Mrs. Clark while he talked to her.

"Mrs. Clark, your EKG is normal, yet you are having some chest pain. We will do some more work-up on you, but is there anything else wrong?"

"I just don't want to live anymore. I am going to die anyway from this cancer, so why suffer?"

Mrs. Clark began to cry and continued, "My niece called me last night and said that she wanted me to leave her everything when I die since she was my only family. She said she would go to court and claim I was incompetent and then become my guardian. That way she could get everything- my house, my car, all of it." "I just can't deal with this. I'd rather die."

The physician replied, "Mrs. Clark, we will do what we can to help. We have already made some arrangements for help and I have asked one of my colleagues to come and talk to you. You get some rest now and we will talk again tomorrow."

The physician was leaving the room as I approached with the medication. He told me of their conversation and asked that I watch her closely today.

"I'll be in my office most of the day today, so call me if anything changes," he stated.

I let Mrs. Clark remain in bed that morning; it would be more beneficial for her to catch up on her rest after the distressing call she had from her niece. It was around 10:00 a.m. when I checked in on her. As I opened the door, I saw Mrs. Clark clutching her chest and gasping for air. I quickly went to her side and opened her airway. Checking for respirations and a pulse and finding neither, I hit the Code button and dialed the hospital operator reporting the cardiopulmonary emergency. The code team and other nurses quickly responded and began resuscitation on Mrs. Clark who was in full arrest. I called out to the unit secretary at the desk to get her doctor. We weren't far into the code when he arrived at her room. Mrs. Clark was not responding to anything being attempted; there were no signs of life.

"Stop the code." her physician announced.

"Are you sure?" asked the emergency room physician who had been leading the code.

"Yes, she has inoperable cancer and there isn't any response to resuscitation."

As the code team departed, Mrs. Clark's physician and I remained at the bedside.

Reflecting on the last day's events in her life and her words that morning, I asked, "Do you think she willed herself to die?"

"That's the only logical conclusion one can draw."

Mrs. Clark was carrying a heavy burden; a burden so great that she couldn't bear it any longer. Although this is an extreme example of the effects of this world's difficulties, there are times that each of us feel that a situation or problem is so great that we cannot hold up to its demands. As nurses, we see a lot of disturbing and devastating situations with our patients. Sometimes, we even tend to take on some these matters and feel overly burdened by these things ourselves. Our Savior offers to carry these burdens for us if we bring them to Him. How many times do we choose to worry and lament about our troubles instead of bringing them to Jesus? We need to spend more time on our knees in prayer than allowing ourselves to be taken to our knees in worry and defeat by the many problems in this world we live. As nurses, we need to also pray for our patients as we minister to their needs. The Lord is faithful in bearing our burdens.

"Cast your burden on the Lord, and He shall sustain you; He shall never permit the righteousness to be shaken."[1]

David Gerstle

Inspiration PRN: Stories About Nurses

GETTING ALONG...
LET'S TRY IT

Why Can't We Play Nice?

Jennifer and Beth were both excellent nurses. They were dependable and competent. They were well liked by their patients and the rest of the staff. Unfortunately, for some reason they could not "stand each other." Put the two together on a shift and you got instant friction. Separate, everyone liked to work with them; but ever together and the staff avoided them at all costs. They would make snide comments about each other, being certain the other heard. Both were natural smilers, but not when they worked together, it was all frowns.

As the unit nurse manager, I made every attempt to avoid scheduling them on the same days as much as possible, however, this didn't work well since both Jennifer and Beth were full-time. I had talked to both of them on a number of occasions about this on-going feud. I explained that they were valued as good nurses, but this dislike for one another was quite a distraction from their otherwise excellent work experience. The nurses vowed each time that they would do better in getting along.

Their resolve to do better did not last long. Jennifer and Beth began their routine during report with a few well-placed put-downs. The other nurses rolled their eyes as they listened; knowing what the rest of the shift was going to be like. All was quiet for a while until Jennifer sat in Beth's "favorite" chair at the nurses' station. Unfortunately, Beth wanted to sit down at the same time as Jennifer.

"That's my chair." Beth said coldly to Jennifer.

"Oh?", Jennifer replied with a touch of sarcasm, "I don't see your name on it."

"Cute," Beth answered curtly, "You know I always sit in *that* chair."

Inspiration PRN: Stories About Nurses

"Well, who made you Queen Bee? Go sit in another chair."

Jennifer turned her back to Beth and became immersed in her charting.

Frustrated and ready to explode, Beth stomped out of the nurses' station. However, it didn't end here. Beth was resolved to win this confrontation. Jennifer eventually had to get up and then Beth could make her move!

The call light comes on from one of Jennifer's patients needing pain medication. Jennifer got up to prepare the medication and then administer it to the patient. Moments later, Beth walks by the nurses' station and sees "her" empty chair. Taking advantage of the moment, she grabs the chair and wheels it down the hall with her to the supply room and puts it in there. She was determined to prevent Jennifer from sitting in it.

Jennifer returns to the station to work on her charting and sees that the chair is missing.

"Where's that chair I was sitting in?" Jennifer asks the unit clerk.

"Beth took it down the hall" the clerk says as she points toward the appropriate hall.

Walking down the hall, Jennifer does not see the chair, but was sure Beth hid it. Being much like Beth, Jennifer first checks the supply room and finds the chair. She rolls it back to the nurses' station and sits down. Beth comes back by and sees Jennifer in her chair. You could literally see smoke coming out of her ears.

The next couple of hours the chair is commandeered by one then the other feuding nurses. The staff are amazed at the conduct of these two middle-aged women. It comes to a critical mass when Beth decides to keep the chair in her possession continuously now. She takes it with her to the patients' rooms. She places one knee on it as she pulls medications from the med cart. She even takes it into the restroom with her.

The charge nurse made attempts to convince these two that their behavior was beyond imagination, but the chair remained hostage. The evening ended with Beth's triumph of keeping the chair the longest.

Of course, as the manager, I received a call the next day from the evening charge nurse about the previous nights' occurrences. She pleaded with me to "do something with those two." That afternoon, Jennifer and Beth were scheduled again. I brought them into my office to discuss the matter. Both knew why they were there and both looked a bit embarrassed. Neither could quite look me in the eye as we sat there.

"I guess you are going to talk to us about last night." Jennifer said as she studied her shoes.

"Yes," pausing for a moment I then continued, "Why can't you two play nice?"

Sheepishly, Beth remarked, "We were pretty stupid last night, huh?"

"Well, it wasn't your greatest moment. Your co-workers weren't very impressed with your professionalism."

Both nurses were genuinely repentant at least for the moment. Each vowed to try to get along with one another. I vowed to motivate them by giving them a second chance to prove themselves instead of immediate discipline for unprofessional behavior.

Sometimes people just don't get along with other people. Personality clashes are often blamed. Habits that are irritating may be the cause of dislike. Whatever the reason, two individuals just don't like each other. If we act upon these feelings of dislike, life itself becomes one big irritation. Everyone around us becomes miserable. One becomes focused on the things this other person does that "bug" us. Our existence is no longer as enjoyable as it once was because we think our "enemy" lives solely to irritate us.

So what can one do?

Jesus has taught us to "love your enemy." As difficult as it is, you must learn to live with people you don't like. Showing kindness when it is not appreciated, listening to others when you don't want to hear them, and spending time with those you don't like are good places to start. Turning selfishness to selflessness when it comes to getting along with others can result in a much happier existence.

"If your enemy is hungry, give him bread to eat; and if he is thirsty, give him water to drink. For so you will heap coals of fire on his head and the Lord will reward you."[1]

David Gerstle

Fight, Fight!

The pager made its presence known by making the all too familiar and irritating Beep, Beep, Beep that reminds you that the shift is always unpredictable for a nursing supervisor and staff. I reached for the pager and punched the button; an emergency page from the hospital operator. As I dialed the operator, I heard her announce over the intercom system the code for security to go to Unit 600. She answered my page a moment later and said, "Dave, there's a fight on the sixth floor! Security should be heading up there now."

"It's not the nurses and doctors fighting, is it?" I asked dryly.

"Very funny! You better get up there." the operator replied while suppressing a laugh.

Sometimes you have to find humor in the stressful environment of the hospital.

Hanging up the phone, I ran to the nearest elevator and quickly caught a ride to the top floor. As I entered the nursing unit, I saw the security officer standing in the hall but no combatants. Some of the nurses were in the nurses' station a bit shook up.

"What's going on?" I asked.

The security officer shrugged his shoulders and said he just arrived himself.

The charge nurse came around the corner and told us the fight had just happened where we were standing but stopped as quickly as it began. According to the charge nurse, one of the fighters was the ex-husband of the patient in room 611 and the other fighter was the current boyfriend of the patient in room 611. The ex-husband came to visit and found the presence of the boyfriend to be a bit more irritating than he could tolerate. A few choice words were exchanged between the two and then a few well-aimed punches were exchanged. The fight progressed from the center of attention's room to the hall.

"The ex is a lot bigger than the boyfriend," the charge nurse continued. "He was really pounding the little guy."

She continued her fight story and explained that the boyfriend was doing the best he could to defend himself, but finally had to retreat. He knew better than to go back toward his girlfriend's room, so he found refuge to the next closest spot; the room next door. Unfortunately, the ex-husband didn't let that interfere with his pugilism. He kept swinging until Boyfriend crawled under the patient's bed. Yes, there was a patient in this room! At this point, Hubby mustered up some intelligence and quickly retreated from the room. Boyfriend stayed right where he was!

"Now you would think our patient in room 612 would have been scared out of his mind." I said while listening to this saga.

"Yes, you would think so," said the charge nurse, "Poor little guy! He has Down's Syndrome and I was sure he would get very upset. But, you know what? He got the biggest kick out of those two guys throwing punches. He was jumping up and down on his bed and yelling at the top of his lungs, "Wrestlin' Oh, boy! Get 'im Get 'im Yeah! Oh boy!"

"Evidently he thinks Wrestlemania has come right to his room, He still has a big grin on his face!" the charge nurse said as she finished her story.

And sure enough she was right! As the security guard and I entered the wrestling fan's room, we found him looking under his bed and grinning at the guy still hiding under his bed.

"Wrestlin' Pow! Pow!" he yelled.

I looked under the bed as well and said, "You can come out now. He's gone."

Boyfriend crawled out, a bit bruised and sporting a nice bright red left eye and a bloody swollen lip. I think his pride hurt more than the rest of him. I sent him off with one of the nurses to get some ice and a little first-aid before we sent him to the ER to be checked out. Next the guard and I went to get the ex-husband. He was now calmed down and very embarrassed.

"I should never have come here. I just lost it. Is that guy all right?" he said.

"Well, he is pretty beat up. The patient in the next room certainly was entertained though," I said.

"I can't believe I did this. Is that patient ok?"

"Yes, he is fine. But you could have hurt him."

"I know, I know!" He shook his head and studied the ground intensely.

I went to check on the other combatant. Boyfriend was holding an ice pack to his eye and was now angry.

"I want to press charges. He had no right to do this to me."

"Well, let me get the security guard and we will call the police. You will have to file charges with them."

"Call them. I'll do it."

I informed the guard and he went to call the police. In the mean time, I took Hubby to a conference room on the unit and let him relax a little. I then told him we had called the police and they would be arresting him. I took a chance that he would not react inappropriately, and he did not. He admitted he was wrong and deserved it. I was thankful that he took it calmly. I really didn't want to provide any more entertainment for the next-door wrestling fan.

Have you ever been so angry that you wanted to beat someone up? So frustrated that you wanted to just pound something or someone until you got it out of your system? I don't think it is only a male problem. Women feel the anger and frustration too. Our humanness wants to get even when we feel wronged. We want to "beat up"

Inspiration PRN: Stories About Nurses

the person who is causing us grief and pain. Sometimes, we also live vicariously through others' actions and revenge toward a common foe. We cheer for the underdog who gets "even" with an oppressor. We sometimes are like the little wrestling fan; Pow, pow, get 'im!

Jesus Christ has taught us a better way to deal with the wrongs others have committed against us. He speaks of turning the other cheek and of walking an extra mile. He teaches us to be kind to our enemies and do good for those that no one else would offer help. This is the opposite of what secular society teaches. We tend to admire those who won't take 'nothin' off of nobody and those who are aggressive and tough. We have a violent society today; it is in the movies, music, and popular books. There is violence in the schools and everyday life. There is terrorism throughout the world. Faith in the safety of flying will never return due to the threat of potential violence in the air. If ever there was justification to seek revenge through violence, the destruction of the World Trade Center would be it. Yet use of force is reserved for the world's governments in answering this cowardly act of terrorism. God has shown us that vengeance is His; we are to live peaceably in our everyday coexistence with others. We must show patience and give up our battles for God to fight. He is all knowing and all-powerful to wage these wars for us.

"If it is possible as much as depends on you, live peaceable with all men. Beloved, do not avenge yourselves, but rather give place to wrath, for it is written, vengeance is mine, I will repay says the Lord."[1]

David Gerstle

THE DUFFS - A FAMILY AFFAIR

The Duffs

There were eight of them. First it was Donny, always smiling and courteous and a delight to have in the nursing program. Donna, a nursing classmate, captured his fancy and after graduation they married making two nurse Duffs.

Two years later, Pat came along, always smiling and courteous, took a liking to nursing classmate, Sandy, and they were married after graduation, making four nurse Duffs. While Pat was in his senior year, mother Duff, Barbara, decided to take nursing. Taking an accelerated curriculum, she graduated just one year behind son Pat, making five nurse Duffs.

Within a few years, Andy, the youngest son, couldn't resist the call to nursing, met Sibby, a nursing classmate, and after graduation they married, making seven nurse Duffs. Before Andy completed his nursing education, father Don lost his job and not knowing what else to do at the time he enrolled in the nursing program. He graduated about a year behind son Andy making eight nurse Duffs all from the same nursing program. A record I am sure.

Even though I did not mention that mother, Andy, and father were smiling and courteous...they were, and much more. The Duffs are portraits of the very essence of Christian service and in the following stories you will see the unique ways God has used them and helped them in their careers.

Here are their stories.

Guardian Angel

Out of sorts for being "pulled" from the Cardiac Care Unit to the medical/surgical floor, Don started his "rounds" in a grumpy mood to assess his assigned patients. The first room he entered was Mr. MacGregor's. Don found him looking over a stack of "Texas Ranger" baseball cards all personally signed; instantly Don's mood changed.

Mac, as he was affectionately called, was an unofficial mascot of the Texas Rangers and Don was a huge fan of this baseball team. Mac had been visiting a patient in the hospital when he had an episode of syncope. He was taken to the Emergency Department. Tests reveal he had suffered a minor myocardial infarction (MI) and was subsequently admitted to the medical/surgical floor for treatment and monitoring.

After assessing Mac, Don continued on his "rounds" and went about providing the necessary nursing care required of his patients. Whenever Don had a break in his duties that evening, he would stop in Mac's room and chat about the Texas Rangers. The next evening, during a break in his Cardiac Care Unit routine, Don took time to go back to visit with Mac; thus began a special friendship.

After Mac's discharge from the hospital, he kept in touch with Don. Mac felt Don's interest in him and friendship contributed to his speedy recovery. Often they went to Texas Ranger games together, for Mac always had an extra ticket to share. The two simply enjoyed each other and had great times just visiting.

Donna, Don's wife, was an emergency room nurse and had taken a few days off to do some things around the apartment with the help of her cousin. Needing some curtain rods, they hurried off to a local hardware store.

After looking over every rod available, they finally made a selection. Just after paying for their purchase they heard someone yell, "We need help over here!" Donna looked around and saw a man lying on the floor. She rushed over and found a man that was "purple" and unconscious. "Call 911," she commanded. Buttons flew everywhere as Donna ripped off the man's shirt to start CPR.

Two breaths...fifteen chest compressions...two breaths...fifteen chest compressions. "I hope those paramedics get here soon," Donna silently prayed. Two breaths...fifteen chest compressions... two breaths fifteen chest compressions. Finally the paramedics arrived, started IV fluids, continued the CPR and rushed the man off to the hospital. Feeling that the man was in good hands now, Donna and her cousin headed for home.

Upon arriving home Don checked out the curtain rods and then asked, "Did you see Mac? He works at the hardware store." "No-oo" Donna answered. Then she told Don about having to provide CPR for a man in the hardware store. "You don't suppose that was Mac, do you?" inquired Don. "I don't think so...but it would have been difficult to tell since the man's face was all purple," replied Donna. "I am going to call the emergency room and just check to see if it was Mac," responded Don. "Yes" it was Mr. MacGregor that had suffered an MI in the hardware store, he was informed. "He is being transferred to the Cardiac Care Unit. It is a good thing someone knew CPR in the store...the physicians say it saved his life. There doesn't appear to be any brain damage and that no doubt is related to his early resuscitation," continued the nurse at the other end of the line, a colleague of Donna's.

Mac had heart bypass surgery and his recovery was surprisingly uneventful. Now he felt he had a special bond with Donna..."she is my guardian angel" he delighted in saying whenever they were together. "Donna is my number one angel and Don is my number two angel."

However, there was one item he regretted, Donna had ripped all the buttons off his shirt and his wife had to sew them back on. "See here, I still have that shirt," Mac would brag pointing to the shirt..."It's a reminder that I know MY guardian angel."

I like to think that when the Psalmist proclaimed, "He (God) will send His angels to take charge and protect you..."[1] that He uses nurses to help accomplish this task. Stories of angels impersonating medical professionals abound...but when nurses are referred to as "angels of mercy" it is the real thing...no impersonation. For everywhere everyday nurses take charge and protect their patients from harm and yes even save lives.

Bonnie Hunt

Doing What Is Right

Pat was looking forward to his 7p—7a shift in the Cardiac Surgical Care Unit. It was Sunday and most of the patients would be about two days post-op and that meant a shift that he could just "cruise" along and enjoy for a change. Upon arriving he discovered that three nurses were scheduled for a low census...four patients. Ugh! And it was his turn to float. Even worse, he had to float to the Medical Intensive Care Unit (MICU) where every patient was on a ventilator, had tubes coming out of every orifice and most were always near death it seemed. With a less than cheerful attitude, Pat shuffled over to MICU and received his assignment. Matters got worse when he was informed that the daughter of Mr. Carter, one of his assigned patients, was allowed to stay at her father's bedside for the night. Silently he fretted, "What happed to the usual rule of the scheduled 'ten-minute' family time."

Right off things were hectic...both of his patients were on ventilators with respiratory problems; both had naso-gastric tubes, both had urinary catheters and both had numerous IV medications that kept him "hopping." Pat was frequently in and out of Mr. Carter's cubicle on one chore or the other, assessing, suctioning, irrigating, turning, and hanging IV medicines. He had little time to speak to the daughter, but even under these less than desirable circumstances, Pat always maintained his professional, competent and caring persona.

Feeling the effects of a strenuous shift, Pat was eagerly preparing to go home, when the daughter of Mr. Carter came out of the cubicle and thanked him for the "good" care he had provided for her dad. Even though Pat appreciated the "thank-you," he was just thankful the shift was over so did not give much thought concerning her comment.

Pat had applied to anesthesia school. About three months after working that "float" shift, he received notice that he was to come in for his interview before the School of Anesthesia board. As would be expected Pat was nervous. The room where the interview was to take place was formal and intimidating. The solemn appearance of the board members as they sat around a large mahogany table did nothing to calm his nerves. The chairman of the board beckoned Pat to take the one lone seat in front of the table. As Pat sat down, he glanced around the table of board members. To his surprise, there sat the daughter who had stayed with Mr. Carter the night he had "floated" to MICU. After both Pat and Mr. Carter's daughter nodded recognition, the interview began. During the intensive questioning, Mr. Carter's daughter made several positive comments on the excellent care Pat had provided her dad.

Trembling hands did not stop Pat from opening the much-anticipated envelope with the return address marked "School of Anesthesia." "I'm accepted, I'm accepted" Pat shouted to any one within earshot. In a few minutes Pat's elation tempered as he acknowledged the comments Mr. Carter's daughter made probably played a big part in his acceptance into anesthesia school. Then he soberly remarked, "You just never know what influence your actions will have."

The first text that came to my mind as Pat related his story to me was "Let your light so shine before men, that they may see your good works..."[1] Then I came across a statement the apostle Paul made in that we all should be mindful of, "We intend to do what is right not only in the Lord's sight, but also in the sight of others."[2]

Bonnie Hunt

God's Answer

Mother Duff, Barbara, told me after graduating she could not shake the question, "Now that I am a nurse God, why am I one? What am I supposed to do?" Not having any clear direction, she took a job in a Pediatric Hospital. Since one of her five children was medically handicapped, she reasoned, "I would be able to understand the parents of medically challenged children."

When nurse son, Andy, heard his mother was going to work with pediatric patients, he presented her with the cleverest "clip on" girl and boy dolls. The clip-on dolls had movable arms, hands and were dressed in the cutest fashion. The girl was dressed in a plaid jumper and white shirt and the boy wore jeans, overalls and a plaid shirt. Barbara treasured these dolls and clipped them on her uniform every evening before leaving for her 11:00 p.m. to 7:00 a.m. shift.

One evening, as Barbara was beginning her shift, she was assigned to admit a child from the children's ER. When the child arrived, accompanied by her mother and grandmother, Barbara was "taken back" at how beautiful this 3 year old was, but oh how pale! The lab report revealed her hemoglobin was 1 gram and blood had been ordered to run though the night.

Sitting on her mother's lap, the child did not even "wince" when the IV was inserted and the blood transfusions started. As Barbara assessed the child frequently, she noted the child barely made any movement, except for changing laps from the mother to the grandmother who themselves appeared to be in a state of shock. Barbara's heart went out to this distraught little family. Toward morning, Barbara observed the transfusions must have done some good;

Inspiration PRN: Stories About Nurses

now instead of white, there was a tinge of pink on the child's face. As she leaned over to listen to her little patient's heart and lungs, the little girl slowly reached out and touched the girl doll clipped on Barbara's uniform. Unclipping the doll from her uniform, Barbara handed it to this precious child. Clutching the doll in her tiny hand, the little patient snuggled closer to her mother and closed her eyes.

Barbara related that she remembers it was 4:45 a.m. when she looked up from her charting and there stood the mother, her lips quivering, inquiring if there was a place she could go and cry. Putting her arm gently around the mother, Barbara quietly ushered her to the nurses' lounge. For reasons she is not sure of, Barbara noted it was 5:55 a.m. when the mother, eyes swollen and red, came out of the nurses' lounge and thanked Barbara for her kindness and then told this story.

She and her daughter, Sarah, had come to visit the grandmother. The grandmother kept saying, "Sarah doesn't look good. You need to take her to see a doctor." Finally they called to make an appointment, "It will have to be the last appointment of the day before the pediatrician could see her," they were told. So late that afternoon they had gone to the pediatrician's office. Confusion and shock set in as they heard words like "Leukemia" "blood transfusions" "helicopter" "St. Judes."

Comforting the mother the best she could, Barbara stayed over from her shift and assisted in transporting the child, who was still clutching that little doll, to the helicopter pad for the ride to St Judes, the nationally known treatment center for childhood cancer. With a promise to keep her and her daughter in her prayers, Barbara bade them farewell and wearily started her trek home. As Barbara looked through the windshield at the bright cloudless morning, she glanced upward and murmured, "God, was last night the reason you wanted me to be a nurse?"

Later at the urging of sons Donny and Pat for Barbara to broaden her nursing experience, she took a job in a Cardiac Care unit. A young woman visiting her father, who had had a myocardial infarction, approached Barbara and inquired, "Do you remember me?" It was the mother of Sarah. Four years had passed and Sarah was in remission and doing great the mother reported. Then she added, "she still cherishes that little doll and I will never forget your kindness in such a distressing experience."

"Everyone who asks will receive, and he who seeks will find, and for those who knock, the door will open."[1]

Bonnie Hunt

While the World Partied

Christmas Eve...the emergency room was raging. Barbara had been called by an agency service to please come and help out. After arriving, it was decided the greatest need was to admit patients from the ER to the medical surgical "floor".

At 11:45 p.m. a mom and dad arrived to the floor holding a frightened, dehydrated, septic young Down's Syndrome child. Needle pricks dotted both hands and arms...souvenirs of unsuccessful intravenous attempts. The physician on call had been notified of the situation. He said not to "stick" the child anymore and that he would come in the next day to insert the intravenous line.

The mom and dad were frantic and to the point of despair. Here it was Christmas Eve; they had other children at home. They didn't know what to do...have the dad go home and "do" Christmas with the children at home and leave mom and ill child at the hospital. Or wait until later the next day when just maybe mom could be there, too. Barbara knew all to well the difficulties a medically handicapped child presents. When asking God, "Why am I a nurse?" Barbara always felt having a medically handicapped child herself would give her a special "edge" in situations like this.

It had only been a few hours since Barbara was feeling sorry for herself. Her grown children were away for the holidays and she and nurse husband Don were scheduled to work. Barbara was "called off" leaving her all alone on Christmas Eve. So she jumped at the chance to work when the agency called and asked her to go to this small county hospital. Her spirit was quickly lifted as she listened to beautiful "soothing" Christmas music during the ride to the hospital. Now facing this child whose temperature was 105 degrees, dehydrated and septic and with no IV access for fluids, her spirit sank as fast as it had risen. "He can't last through the night without intravenous fluids," she reasoned. Assessing the child, Barbara saw a vein in his foot that just maybe would hold an intravenous needle. She decided to call the physician back and tell him that she did see a vein in the child's foot that might be accessed. While waiting for the physician to come to the phone, Barbara said she could hear a lot of gaiety...Christmas music playing, lively conversation, children squealing with delight, and the clinking of glasses and clanging of dishes; it seemed a good time was being had by all. When the physician finally came to the phone, Barbara informed him of the vein in the child's foot. After a long hesitation the physician finally said "o.k., but only one stick."

Barbara immediately marched to the closest bathroom, fell to her knees and pleaded, "God you know the desperate situation this little boy is facing; he needs fluids and antibiotics now. I can't do this but you can! Amen." Quietly gathering the IV fluid, tubing and 22-gauge angiocath, Barbara approached the frightened child. Explaining to the mom and dad the importance of not letting the boy move his foot, Barbara inserted the needle and immediately got a "flashback" then taped the site securely and started the fluids and antibiotic.

With the IV infusing without difficulty and the first dose of the IV antibiotic completed, Barbara busied herself admitting several more patients transferred from the ER. As the "mad house" quieted down, Barbara went to check on the little Down's Syndrome patient. Stepping into the room she noticed the mother had finally "let go" and had fallen sound asleep. Barbara took an extra blanket that was in the room and gently covered up the weary mother. As she paused at the door of the room and glanced back at the scene of this mother all-alone in the room with a very ill handicapped child on Christmas Eve, she thought, "what a contrast to the merriment she had heard in the home of the physician she had talked to earlier that night. And how like the night Jesus was born. Mary, weary and alone, in a cattle stall with her first born Son 'using an animal's feeding trough for His cradle' while the rest of the world partied."

Bonnie Hunt

God I Need You Again!

Intensive Care Unit...young man...quadriplegic...tracheostomy...septic...arms and legs so edematous no site for an intravenous could be found...waiting for a physician to insert a subclavian line. In walks Barbara...fear staring at her...fear of a collapsed lung...fear of chest tubes...fear of dying. A previous experience had set the stage for fear to play its havoc. It was like "déjà vu". On this young quadriplegic's last admission to ICU he needed intravenous fluids and no peripheral site for an IV could be located, so a subclavian line had been ordered...resulting in nicked lung...pneumothorax...chest tubes...one scared patient. Ever compassionate Barbara thought, "there has to be some way a peripheral IV line can be started to avoid the trauma of a subclavian access." She found a quiet spot and prayed, "Lord, I need your help. I can not do this without you." Then she reminded the Lord of the incident with the young Down's patient that also had no accessible IV site and He helped her to access a vein in his foot. Barbara recalled one of her nurse sons telling her, "In difficult situations, you can usually find good veins in the upper arms." Collecting fluids, tubing and a 22-gauge angiocath Barbara set about to start an IV in a very edematous arm where she could not see or feel a vein. Without using a tourniquet, Barbara inserted the 22-gauge angiocath in the young man's upper arm where she thought a vein should be and got an immediate "flashback"...now we had one relived patient...one relieved nurse...and a "Thank you Lord."

"With God, nothing is impossible."[1]

Bonnie Hunt

Another Guarding Angel

"Please! Please! Let's go to that Japanese restaurant where they prepare the food in front of you and throw knives up in the air," pleaded Zack. It had been a long and tiring day for grandmother Barbara and Uncle Don shepherding the grandkids to dental appointments, school uniform shopping and a late afternoon ball game. The grandkids were also tired and hungry. When Uncle Don asked, "Where would you all like to eat?" Zack piped up immediately. It was late and passed the first seating for the Kanpai of Tokyo restaurant, so Uncle Don tried to suggest other alternatives like Taco Bell. No takers.

The lateness of the hour did not dampen Zack and his cousins' enthusiasm for a knife throwing Japanese dinner and they all agreed it was worth the wait when they were ushered to a table right up front for a first hand view of the food preparation. Shortly after being seated, a lady close by started up a conversation with Barbara. The lady explained that her 11-year-old daughter was to have back surgery for her scoliosis the next day (Friday) and she was treating her daughter to this special dinner. As they continued to chat, Barbara sensed that both Mother and daughter were anxious and scared about the upcoming surgery.

"Your daughter's name doesn't happen to be Ashton?" Barbara inquired.

Startled the mother replied, "Why yes! How did you know?" Barbara explained that at her Monday night Bible Study group the pastor's daughter had requested prayer for her friend, Ashton, who was to have surgery for her scoliosis in a few days and "I just wondered if your daughter might be the Pastor's daughter's friend." Now sensing that this was more then just a coincidence

Inspiration PRN: Stories About Nurses

Barbara continued, "We prayed for Ashton this past Monday evening." Barbara then introduced her self as a Registered Nurse and offered her services if they needed her.

Monday was a day for errands. While mulling over in her mind the list of chores she needed to accomplish and thinking how thankful she was to have a much needed day off, Barbara glanced out the window of her car and noticed the children's hospital exit. Suddenly Barbara found herself making a quick U-turn and heading for the hospital...giving into a strong impression she should visit Ashton and see how she was doing.

Entering Ashton's room, Barbara found her all alone and moaning in pain. Upon making inquiries at the nurses' station, Barbara was told that Aston's Mother had gone home to shower and change clothes since she had spent the weekend at Aston's bedside. "Is it all right if I sit with her for a while?" With the request granted Barbara headed back to Ashton's room where she found her still crying out in pain and said she needed to use the bedpan. Ashton had been too "out of it" to push the Patient Control Analgesia (PCA) pump that was to help control her pain. So Barbara pushed the button and helped Ashton on and off the bedpan, which took some special maneuvering to avoid further injury to her spine. After Barbara pushed the PCA pump button several more times to help relieve her pain, Ashton's frail little body seemed to relax.

"I have orders to get Ashton up," informed the physical therapist entering the room. Barbara objected, "There is no way Ashton will be able to get up with all the pain she has been experiencing." "I have orders for her to be out of bed today," insisted the therapist. Quietly Barbara awaked Ashton and told her the therapist was here to get her up out of bed. "No! I can't do it," whimpered Ashton. With great difficulty and much moaning and groaning from Ashton the therapist and

Barbara got her out of bed and in a chair. Ashton was too groggy to be left alone, so Barbara stayed and held her hand and then helped the therapist get her back to bed. As Barbara was helping the therapist return Ashton back to her bed, she thought to herself she was sure God had impressed her to come visit Ashton, for there was no way the therapist could have gotten Ashton out of bed and back alone.

Once back to bed Ashton drifted off in a daze while Barbara continued to gently stroke her hand to let her know someone was still by her side. Some two and half hours later the grandparents showed up inquiring, of Barbara, "Who are you?" After a brief explanation Barbara left to finish her errands.

Barbara Duff insists that her nursing career has had its many rewards...but the one she cherishes the most is the following:

Barbra,

I'm sorry it has been so long for me to write you. In fact you probably do not even remember me. I had spine surgery and the night before I met you at Kanpi (Kanpai) of Tokyo. As I laid on the hospital bed, I remember just wanting to undo the surgery I went through. PAIN was all I felt and I was nothing but miserable. Then I remember awaking to a tender hand holding on to mine, telling me it was alright, that God was with me. You are hazy in my mind almost like a person I dreamt, like an ANGEL!! That is how I will always think of you, my Guardian Angel. After you coasted (coaxed) me to sit up for the first time, you told me what a great job I had done. My family was gone out to eat, I had no one except you. Last thing I remember was you holding my hand and then I fell asleep. When I awoke you were gone like an Angel. Thank you, for being so caring, so extrodary (extraordinary), so wonderful, as to come and visit a person you did not know. Forever, I know, I will remember you. My Angel.

Thank you,
Ashton Teska

God works in mysterious ways to "Send His angels to take charge and protect you..."[1] And that angel just might be Barbara Duff.

Bonnie Hunt

Acknowledgments

David's stories for the most part are drawn from his experiences during the fifteen years he spent in clinical practice prior to his teaching career. Bonnie's stories come from a variety of sources...relatives, friends, colleagues, students and her own experiences. Also, some of the ideas for her stories have come from clips of articles that she read or that were passed along to her for inspirational thoughts to share with the students over the last 26 years. Most of these thoughts are not from "hard" copies of material but memories that have stayed with her over the years. If a hard copy does exist, it is worn, faded and dog-eared with only the author's name...no source indicated. A diligent effort has been made to give proper credit in the following acknowledgments. If she has over looked giving proper credit to anyone, please accept her apologies. If you contact her at Post Office Box 423, Collegedale, Tennessee, 37315, corrections will be made prior to additional printings. With a few exceptions, "real" names of those involved in the stories, or those sharing their stories, have been used with their permission.

Bible texts are quoted from the New King James (NKJ) and from the Clear Word (CW).

"Jesus Prays with Us"	[1] Desire of Ages, p.667.
"Near Misses"	[1] James 5:16.
"Can We Pray?"	[1] 1Thessalonians 5:17.
	[2] James 5:16.
"Atheist Prayer"	[1] John 1:12.
"Just a Nurse?"	The introductory scene was inspired by a story retained in memory.
	[1] Matthew 4:23.
	[2] 1 Corinthians 12: 5, 9.

Inspiration PRN: Stories About Nurses

"CATS, PETS, and MRIs Don't Supply the Care; Nurses Do". The title and the tribute to nurses were excerpted from an article by Linda Chitwood- source unknown.

	[1] Galatians 5:9.
"Life is Backwards"	[1] Editorial by Laura Billings, St. Paul Pioneer Press May 2001
	[2] Matthew 6:33.
	[3] Matthew 22:37.
	[4] Matthew 6:31.
"No Brains, All Brawn"	[1] Hebrews 4:16.
"The Name is Nurse, Male Nurse!"	
	[1] Colossians 3:17.
"Too Busy to Help"	[1] 1 John 3:17.
"First Clinical Jitters"	[1] Matthew 7:12.
"Gifts Differing"	[1] Romans 12:7-11.
"Singing Nurse Assistant"	[1] "Jesus Loves Me" William B. Bradbury, 1892.
	[2] "Sweet By and By" J.P. Webster, 1860.
	[3] "This Little Light of Mine" arrg. by Alma Blackmon, 1984.
	[4] Matthew 7:12.
"A Bedpan by Any Other Name"	
	[1] Titus 3-5.
"Windy Wake-Up Call"	[1] John 3: 5-8.
"Living Water"	[1] John 4:14.

"Good Medicine" The following were gleaned from the Journal of Nursing Jocularity. The Humor Magazine for Nurses. "A patient rang his call light..." V.7 #3 Fall 1997. "A nursing assistant tells..." V.8 #2 Summer 1998. "An ER nurse tells..." V.6 #2 Summer 1996. "Mark was born with one ventricle..." V.7 #3 Fall 1997. "Art Linkletter tours a nursing home..." V.3 #4 Winter 1993.

[1] Proverbs 17:22.

"The Healing Word"   [1] Psalms 107:20.

Inspiration PRN: Stories About Nurses

"Christmas Code Blue"	[1] Ezekiel 37:26.
"Dismayed"	[1] Deuteronomy 31:8.
"Unusual? Maybe Not"	[1] Jeremiah 29: 11.
	[2] Isaiah 41:10.
"Promises"	[1] Jeremiah 29:11.
	[2] 1 Peter 5:7.
"Never Give Up!"	[1] James 5:15.
"Disillusioned"	[1] Matthew 19: 26.
	[2] Galatians 5:9.
"Body Image Aerobics"	[1] Psalms 27:14
	[2] Isaiah 41:10.
"Ain't Gonna Do It!"	[1] Isaiah 35: 3, 4.

"Florence" Some of the content came from memory; other aspects of the content came from an article that came across my desk "Florence Nightingale Becomes a Nurse" by Paul Chrastina - source unknown.

[1] Romans 8:28.

"A Train with No Caboose"- originally published in Adventist Review, April 16, 1998.

"Jumping to Conclusions"	[1] Matthew 7:1.
"Instructions"	[1] Psalms 32:8.
"Don't Run"	[1] Psalms 40:1
	[2] Psalms 37: 23, 39.
"Painful Lessons"	[1] Matthew 11:28-30.

"How Will I Know I "m Hurting?" As told by Nettie Gerstle.

[1] 1 John 1:9.

"Painful Confusion"	[1] Psalms 55:22.
"Solving the Wrong Problem"	[1] Psalms 110: 119.
"Out of the Darkness"	[1] Matthew 11:29,30.
"CCU Madness"	[1] Psalms 51:10,11.
"Left to Die"	[1] Proverbs 18:24.
"The Way Home"	[1] Isaiah 42:16.
	[2] Matthew 6:33.
	[3] Isaiah 30:21.
"Plans"	[1] Psalms 36:5.
	[2] Psalms 37:4.

Inspiration PRN: Stories About Nurses

"Though I walk through the valley of the shadow of death..."
                            [1] Proverbs 14:32
                            [2] 1 Corinthians 15:51,52.

"A New Beginning"   [1] Matthew 14:1-3.
"Will to Live, Will to Die"   [1] Psalms 55:22.
"Why Can't We Play Nice?" [1] Proverbs 25:21,22.
"Fight, Flight"   [1] Romans 12:18,19.

The Duffs. A special acknowledgment to the "Duffs", Barbara, Don, Donna, and Pat for so generously and enthusiastically sharing their stories.

"Guardian Angel"   [1] Psalms 91:11.
"Doing What Is Right"   [1] Matthew 5:16.
                            [2] 2 Corinthians 8:21.
"God's Answer"   [1] Luke 11:10.
"God I Need You Again!"   [1] Luke 1:37.
"Another Guardian Angel" [1] Psalms 91:11.

About the Authors

David S. Gerstle, Ph.D., R.N. and Bonnie C. Hunt, M.S.N., R.N. are professor and professor emeritus, respectively, in the School of Nursing on the campus of Southern Adventist University in Collegedale, Tennessee. Together, they have over 49 years of nursing experience. The stories in this book are based on their clinical practice and teaching careers.